1996

Profit Fever

Profit Fever

The Drive to Corporatize
Health Care and
How to Stop It

Charles Andrews

Common Courage Press   Monroe, Maine

Library of Congress Cataloging-in-Publication Data

Andrews, Charles, 1947-
Profit fever: the drive to corporatize health care
and how to stop it/Charles Andrews.
p. cm.
Includes bibliographical references and index.
ISBN 1-56751-056-6 (pbk.).
ISBN 1-56751-057-4 (cloth)
1. National health insurance--United States. 2. Health care
reform--United States. 3. Medical care--United States--
Finance. 4. Medical corporations--United States. 5. Insurance,
Health--California. 6. Health care reform--California. I. Title.

| RA412.5.U6A69 1995 | 95-14883 |
| 338.4'33621'0973--dc20 | CIP |

Common Courage Press
Box 702
Monroe, ME 04951
Call or write for free catalog
207-525-0900   fax: 207-525-3068

First Printing

Contents

338.433621
A562

156,353

Preface

In the United States, the last advanced industrial country that leaves health insurance in the hands of corporate capital, most people either have a horror story of medical disaster and financial ruin in their family, or they know someone else's suffering at the hands of an insurance company, a managed care health plan, or just generally a heartless society whose economic powers knocked a person down and then said, you're on your own.

The insurance business affects more than health. Whether people get health care through employment, from social insurance, or by expense out of pocket can decide whether they change jobs and their strength when they negotiate their pay. The consequences extend to marriage and divorce and to security in old age.

People are looking around and noticing that twists in their individual lives are not an accident of fate but a common problem. They have formed a movement to obtain health care as a right. Furthermore, on a political landscape where it seems no section of society has a banner for working people as a whole, the single payer movement may awaken people to fundamental questions of social change.

This book has two purposes. First, it gives an account of the forces that developed medicine from a set of professions into a corporatized industry. With this perspective the reader can understand news reports about the economics and politics of health reform.

Second, the book explains the single payer plan—health care without insurance companies—and tells the story of a mass movement for it, the voter-initiated California Health Security Act. As Proposition 186, it failed to pass in Nov. 1994, but anyone interested in health reform can learn much from the Act and the drive to pass it. This writer was an active participant in the campaign.

Although this is a book of political economy, there is no unexplained technical talk here. All it says is that we are not doing a policy study. Political economy recognizes the conflict between economic interests, while policy studies imagine there is one common goal. They evade conflicts or pretend that they can be resolved to the roughly equal benefit of all parties. It isn't so.

Thanks go to Steve Schear, who welcomed a stranger into the California single payer campaign even if he could foresee later disagreement over strategy; and Harold and Anne Fox, Alan Hanger, Tom Condit, and Don Bechler, who supported an ancestor of this book because they want activists to study and think. These people and Dan Cloak, Lucinda Dutcher, Ted Kalman, Vishu Lingappa, and Alex Pappas, plus many others, gave the book extensive input. I also thank all the other helpful persons who united in the California campaign. They are different from each other, proving that good people come in every variety.

1

How Health Care Became a Problem

Insurance for medical bills was born in the United States in the 1930s. It was due neither to commercial insurance companies nor to physicians, who were the supreme economic power in the health field.

A 1930 survey found that only one million of 35 million workers had any coverage for nonoccupational ailments. Half of them were employed by railroads, which had made arrangements for care of their mobile workers since the middle of the nineteenth century. The other 97% of the nation's work force had nothing.[1]

Blue Cross Hospital Insurance

On Jan. 1, 1930, Baylor University Hospital in Dallas, Texas created a plan for public school teachers. In return for a fee of six dollars per year, Baylor guaranteed the teacher up to three weeks of care in a semi-private room when her physician ordered hospitalization. Baylor created the plan after it examined unpaid bills and found that many of the delinquent patients were teachers. By 1935, 23,000 people from 400 employee groups had enrolled.

No middleman stood between Baylor and the insured workers. In 1932, seven nonprofit hospitals in Sacramento, California, joined together and made an offer similar to the one in Dallas. They created a nonprofit health insurance company to administer their plan.

Although the hospitals were nonprofit, they depended on revenue from a steady stream of patients. The fixed costs of bonds and overhead had to be met, and the occupancy ratio was a matter of vital concern to the hospital owners and executives. Large numbers of employees collected in cities, but most were unable to save enough money for a severe illness or injury. In the 1920s, the automobile companies had found a way to sell their big-ticket item—installment credit. With the onset of the Depression, hospitals faced a decline in revenue while costs rolled on. Insurance plans were their solution. From the beginning in Texas, the plans became known as Blue Cross and grew rapidly.

Blue Cross Enrollment (millions)[2]

1937	1.3
1939	4
1945	15
1948	30
1951	37
1960	60

The initiative for Blue Cross insurance came from hospitals. Physicians were uneasy about it. Traditionally, the medical doctor kept a direct relationship with each individual or family. The physician treated the sick based on their ability to pay a fee. The patient had no professional knowledge or group resource with which to evaluate the doctor's diagnosis and treatment. True, many physicians balanced the needs and financial abilities of their better off and impoverished patients. These were the days when doctors even made house calls, carrying all the implements of their trade in a black bag. The physician knew his patients by name, often from one generation to the next.

Still, doctors were in business for themselves, neither employees nor an employer, except perhaps for a nurse or assistant. Organized in powerful local medical societies and governing themselves with the sanction of state authority through licensing boards, physicians were the unchallenged economic power of medicine.

New Forms of Health Insurance
Hospital insurance was popular and was extended to other parts of health care. Surgeons tended to see the trend of things. Unlike the gen-

eral practitioner who performs almost all his work in his office or at the patient's home, the surgeon needs the resources of a hospital. In 1939 the Michigan State Medical Society started a plan that covered the fees of surgeons and other hospital-based specialists. In one year it enrolled 60,000 workers at Ford Motor Company. This was the birth of Blue Shield.

Physicians made sure they governed Blue Shield. They controlled the board of directors and set up the plan with close ties to the medical society. They defined the fee schedule.

Blue Shield limited benefits to conditions treated in a hospital, leaving the relationship between a patient and a primary care doctor in his office undisturbed. The fees were defined by procedure, so much for an appendectomy, so much for setting a bone, etc. A doctor could charge whatever amount he liked; the patient was liable for any excess over Blue Shield's coverage. However, doctors pledged to accept the fee as payment in full if the patient's income was less than $2,000 (or $2,500 for a family).

By the end of 1941, the Michigan plan enrolled 450,000 members. Such plans remained local or statewide, but they unified their rules and authorized the national Blue Shield logo in 1946. Enrollment grew right behind Blue Cross. In 1950 there were 15 million members of Blue Shield plans; in 1962, the number was 56 million.

A historian of medical economics observes, "The early success of the Blue Cross plans proved the biggest surprise to those organizations which up to that time thought they were the last word on everything called insurance—the private insurance companies."[3] By the early 1930s they had written group health policies for about 30,000 people; Metropolitan Life wrote a plan for General Motors in 1928. In the mid-thirties the insurance corporations decided to follow the Blue Cross lead. Their hospital insurance also set limits to benefits and had no intention of covering the full cost of treatment. The businesses to whom they sold their plans liked this feature. The insurance company custom-designed a package for each employer, who decided how much coverage his employees should get.

An employer whose plan appeared generous could demand extra commitment and effort from his workers in return. On the other hand, employers offering little or no health care kept their costs down. In general, companies enjoyed the option of how to relate to their labor force, an advantage they would lose if a universal system guaranteed everyone the health care she needs.

For sharp business reasons, a number of commercial insurance companies and a multitude of employers created the endless variety of rules and clauses that plague doctors, hospitals and patients today. Enrollment in commercial insurers' group hospital plans grew from 8.5 million in 1944 to 57 million in 1961.[4]

When the United States entered World War II in 1941, the wartime command economy finally pulled the U.S. out of the Depression. There was an extreme labor shortage, and the federal government imposed wage stabilization rules. In order to attract and retain employees, companies forbidden to raise money wages granted health benefits instead. From 1941 to 1945 the percentage of the population with some form of health insurance, mostly limited to hospital bills, rose to approximately 25%.[5]

In the later 1940s the insurance companies added individual policies to their product line. If your employer did not provide benefits or you were in business for yourself, and you had the money, you could buy coverage. By 1951, commercial insurance companies, in group and individual hospital plans, surpassed Blue Cross. By 1961, 800 companies sold individual policies to 40 million customers.

Over time Blue Cross added new charges and exclusions to its plans, becoming more like the commercial insurance companies.

Many large corporate employers self-insure. They might contract with an insurance company for administrative services. In recent years they have signed up with managed care plans, too, in an effort to restrain cost increases.

After the steady growth of hospital insurance through the Depression, World War Two, and the 1950s, the Social Security Administration reported in 1961 that such insurance covered about 60% of private expenditures for hospital care.[6]

Insurance for hospital bills and even for the bill from the doctor who performs an operation is not comprehensive health insurance. A comprehensive policy covers all the services used in a treatment.

In 1961, insurance coverage was spotty and extremely unequal. One person in four (26%) had no health insurance of any kind. Policies covering the other 74% went only a little way toward paying the bill: 27% of the $21 billion that Americans spent privately for personal health care passed through insurance organizations. Coverage might be group or individual, with a profit or nonprofit company, and paid by employer or employee or split in some ratio between them. Exclusions, limits, copayments and deductions were more numerous than holes in Swiss cheese. The situation was much worse for persons age 65 and over; two out of three had no hospital insurance.[7]

Cooperatives and Union Services

Although health insurance devoted to business purposes, if not always explicitly run for profit, dominated the field with their tens of millions of customers, a persistent exceptional trend developed in opposition to commercial models.

In 1929 a Farmers' Union in the poor area around Elk City, Oklahoma started what is believed to be the first genuine medical cooperative in the United States. Members paid an admission fee, annual dues, and some charges for X-rays and hospital stays. As a group, they had the nerve to employ doctors for a salary. The members received full care for their ailments rather than drawing on a set dollar amount per procedure. In contrast to the physician-ruled Blue plans, the members elected the board of directors on the principle of one enrollee, one vote. To the credit of the nobler side of the medical profession, Michael Shadid, a socially conscious physician who immigrated from Syria when he was a child, was a key organizer of the Elk City cooperative.

For twenty years the local medical society and the AMA tried everything to kill the Elk City group, but they failed.[8] It and similar cooperatives had to fight legal battles with local medical societies. The organized physicians, drawing on the power they had through their instrument of self-regulation, the state licensing board, tried to make life impossible for doctors who worked with cooperative plans. The medical society even kept them from entering hospitals. Courts eventually ruled against these tactics.

Yet by 1961, there were only 150,000 people in cooperative plans across the United States.

Trade unions occasionally took on the job of providing health benefits. In 1913 in New York City, the International Ladies' Garment Workers Union established the first union-run medical center. In the early 1950s, the United Mine Workers started its own network of clinics. This service, too, was an exception, set up for a scattered, rural industry with specialized health problems and run by a single union dealing with a large number of mostly small employers.

Health Maintenance Organizations

A health maintenance organization (HMO) goes beyond an insurance plan. In one way or another it blends insurance and the provision of treatment itself. In the purest form, the HMO owns and operates its medical care facilities; contracts with hospitals are common, too.

In 1933 Henry Kaiser contracted with a physician-entrepreneur to run a clinic that would repair his isolated workers pouring cement for the Grand Coulee Dam. This was a prepaid service. As a steel mill owner and ship builder, Kaiser started an HMO in 1942 at his shipyards in Richmond, California, across the Bay from San Francisco. The HMO retained a staff of doctors on salary or other financial terms; they worked in the HMO's clinics and centers. Kaiser did not have to build its facilities. The federal government paid the construction cost during World War Two for clinics in the San Francisco Bay Area and other locations. After the war, the Kaiser Hospital Foundation bought them at the giveaway price of one cent on the dollar.

The Kaiser system grew to be a mighty force in northern and southern California. This happened not only because it was popular but out of conscious decision by the top executives. Although formally nonprofit, the Kaiser Plan runs on typical business principles. The administrators noted that if they kept a static roster of clients, the average age would gradually increase, raising costs and demands for service. Therefore, Kaiser aimed for as many decades as it could to bring in waves of new enrollees who would keep the average age from rising.[9]

Kaiser remained an exception until health maintenance organizations took off in the 1970s and 1980s. As long as physicians had the economic role and the clout to dominate medicine on the basis of fee for service, HMOs could not become a common method of organizing health care.

Racism Prior to the Black Upsurge

In 1950, a few years before the civil rights movement burst forth, two medical schools in the United States trained black physicians. Only one doctor in 50 was African-American. Almost all were general practitioners, because only 105 black physicians had been allowed to complete graduate specialist programs; of these, ten served the entire South. Hospitals almost entirely refused to allow black surgeons and other doctors to treat patients at their facilities. At mid-century, the life expectancy of African-American people was ten years less than that for whites. The infant mortality rate was 55% higher. (Those were the good old days. Today the black rate for infant mortality rate is 2.2 times that of white newborns.)[10]

Women's Labor in Health Care

A boy grows up to become a doctor; a girl becomes a nurse. This was an almost universal rule until recently, and it is still more true than not.

If the phrase "nurse's office" was not simply nonsense in comparison with "doctor's office," it referred to a shabby corner located in a hospital, a private home of the well-to-do, or a public health office. In the nineteenth century, hospitals were charity or religious institutions, and their nurses were badly paid. Some nurses worked in private homes, where they were on call 24 hours a day, treated like servants, and paid mostly with room and board.

The history of nursing intersects the history of public health. The latter (endorsed in 1893 by Florence Nightingale under the term "health nursing") began as part of the minimum social response needed to protect the upper classes from epidemics jumping out of slum streets that were "dirty, filled with vegetable and animal refuse, without sewers or gutters, but supplied with foul, stagnant pools instead."[11]

Nurses and other women were sent to the homes of the lower income levels of the working class. They treated victims of infectious disease and taught disease prevention and child nutrition.

While public health nurses were women, the state boards were typically run by medical doctors from private practice, men who knew little or nothing about public health. In California, physicians made up the Board of Public Health by law, and the directors were drawn from private practice.[12] Under their official neglect, resources for public health were extremely scarce and remain so.

The public health movement had its weaknesses, like a tendency to bring their good works to the poor as a gift from above. It needs to change with circumstances, too. Some people thought its job was done once communicable diseases were largely wiped out, but the public health approach of working with the entire population before acute disease develops remains valid. It must simply be practiced in new ways. However, the organization of medicine as a business, treating individuals with specific ailments for a price, made it impossible for public health to develop along with increasing medical and scientific knowledge into what it should be: a major part of how we as a society prevent and quickly detect illness. The numbers of public health nurses by the 1920s peaked at one per 10,000 people. Meanwhile, physicians, although keeping themselves scarce by methods of professional monopoly, were in supply at a ratio of one per 730 persons in 1920 (down to one per 800 by 1930).[13]

Public health nurses, and women in health care generally, have been the unrewarded, almost underground representatives of the ways that we should organize effective health care for society as a whole.

Medical Care for the Aged

While working Americans had more or less health insurance, and although county and other government-run hospitals treated the poor at least in emergencies, the health needs of the aged were not addressed until the 1960s. At the start of the decade, more than half (53%) of the people age 65 and over had no health insurance. In 1961 the average private health care expense of aged persons was 80% more than that for the population as a whole, and insurance paid only one-sixth of it.[14] The struggle to win the program for the aged that we know today as Medicare is a political lesson in how conservative economic groups resist liberal solutions for social problems. It goes back to 1935, when Social Security was passed. There had been calls to meet the health needs of the aged as well as to assure them a public pension. However, President Roosevelt's study group, the Committee on Economic Security, held back its report on health insurance until after Congress passed the Social Security Act, out of fear that doctors and insurance companies would kill the entire bill.[15] (Another compromise excluded farm workers from Social Security.) The dominant economic force in medicine at that time, the physicians of the American Medical Association, even defeated a clause authorizing the Social Security Board merely to conduct a study of the health care problem.

FDR's study group on medical care proposed a liberal scheme rather than a radical democratic plan, let alone a socialist idea. Like Social Security itself, financing went through the employer. In this case, employers would receive tax credits for their health insurance contributions. General tax revenues would be called upon only to help states treat the poor. The concept of a multi-tier health system is an old one.

Senator Robert Wagner of New York accepted the liberal framework and introduced legislation in 1939, retaining the idea of a federal-state scheme. Four years later Wagner offered a bill for a straight national program. In the 1945 version of the bill, financing copied the regressive pattern set by Social Security: employer and employee would each pay 1.5% of the first $3,600 of wages. After President Roosevelt's death in 1945, Harry Truman supported national health insurance.

It should be noted that in 1942, a liberal group of doctors, the Physicians Forum, organized nationally and favored health insurance for the aged paid through Social Security. They later supported the Wagner proposal.

Employers and physicians denounced national health insurance as socialized medicine, although no one ever wrote a major bill based on financing through progressive taxation, uniform benefits for all, and government-run or nonprofit clinics staffed by physicians on salary. Even these features do not add up to a socialist solution. For example, government would still buy pills from drug companies.

Hospital administrators as well as the Public Health Service refused to support national health insurance. In 1950 the American Medical Association outspent the group in favor of the plan by $2.25 million to $36,000, financing a smear campaign by the reactionary public relations firm Whitaker and Baxter.

In 1951 Truman abandoned the fight for national insurance. He retreated to advocating health insurance for the aged under Social Security. Twenty-one years later, the Kennedy administration submitted a bill for health insurance for the aged. It failed by three votes in the Senate.

Medicare: One Era Closes, Another Begins
Medicare for the aged along with the smaller Medicaid program for the poor was passed in July 1965. The AMA spent $7 million to defeat it but failed. One reason was that Blue Cross and the American Hospital Association (AHA) supported the legislation because it had goodies for them that we will describe later.[16]

Medicare was the last wave in a tide of liberal reform that had begun at the turn of the century with the Progressive movement of upper middle class people. It reached a climax with Social Security and other New Deal programs. Like the New Deal, Medicare was enacted at a time of unrest and struggle—the one during the Great Depression and the industrial union drive, the other during the 1960s anti-racist movement and the protest against U.S. war on Vietnam. Social Security was perhaps FDR's most solid domestic achievement, as was Medicare for Lyndon Johnson. Strangely, they were off to the side from the main battles of the day. They were partial solutions. With their shortfall of benefits, less than progressive financing, and other institutional defects, these programs contained the seeds of new problems. Yet no one would deny that Social Security, and Medicare with Medicaid, raised the minimum level of human decency that people of every political stripe honor in word if not in action.

The passage of Medicare left old shortcomings like incomplete and unequal insurance coverage. Today the program is riddled with extra charges: a deductible of $652 against the first 60 days of hospital care; 20% copayment of a doctor's allowed fees; another 20% if the doctor decides to bill it; and no payment for prescription drugs outside the hospital.

In addition, institutional changes made by Medicare itself combined with deep economic trends to produce new problems, troubles that have built up to the health care crisis of 1994.

2

Medicine Goes Corporate

Spending on health care has risen steadily since World War II. From less than 4% of the economy in 1950, health now takes 14%.

Personal Consumption Expenditures (percent of total)[17]

	1950	1960	1970	1980	1990
Medical care	3.6	5.0	7.2	9.5	14.0
Motor vehicles and parts	7.1	6.0	5.6	5.2	5.4

Part of the spending growth is a change in economic focus that happens in all developed countries. Market demand and technological advantage shift from one industry to another. In the case of the health business, technical change has not reduced costs, for reasons examined later. In 1929, medical care took 3.5% of the gross national product.[18] By 1960, health care spending had risen toward 6% of gross domestic product in the United States, Canada, Germany, Japan, and the United Kingdom; by 1990 these countries were in the 6% to 9% range—except the United States, which spent over 12% on health care.[19]

Because the medical industry was growing, sellers who enjoyed various forms of exclusive positions as suppliers (physicians, hospitals, drug and equipment companies) could raise prices more than the average for the economy. The table above shows dollar figures. Real care given to the population lags in an inflationary setting. (Similarly, the declining percentage of motor vehicles in expenditures does not mean that automobiles became cheaper. Over the last twenty years, prices measured by the number of weeks' pay required to buy a car have increased. However, people keep their vehicles longer.)

Another reason for the growth of health spending is actually a phase in the fall of living standards for working people. The decline started in the late 1960s and continues to this day. By 1992, workers' average weekly earnings had 14% less purchasing power than in 1970. In 1967, 45% of new jobs paid less than $13,600 (in 1980 dollars); from then to 1984, two-thirds of the new jobs offered less than this amount. In just two years of so-called economic recovery, 1991 to 1993, median family income adjusted for inflation fell 3%.[20]

While wages adjusted for inflation stagnated and fell, employee health plans improved for a decade or so. Each employer could boast to his workers about the specific features in his benefit package, which is harder to compare with other companies than money wages. Trade unions too weak to win pay increases went along with the tendency to substitute improvement in benefits.

To a small degree, tax treatment of benefits versus wages encouraged this trend. A wage increase bumped up Social Security and income taxes; better medical coverage did not. However, we should not overestimate the impact of tax rules. In 1979, the $14 billion that they cost federal and state governments was less than 10% of spending on health care.[21]

The fundamental development is the fall in the standard of living for the majority of people. In the 1980s, benefits joined wages in decline. From 1983 to 1993 the percentage of workers with employer-provided health coverage fell from 66% to 61%.[22] Those still holding onto insurance paid higher copayments and deductibles.

Another reason for the growth of health care spending was the specific form of Medicare as legislated in 1965. President Lyndon Johnson and Congressman Wilbur Mills horse-traded their way to passage of Medicare. Hospitals supported it after they were assured that Blue Cross would process their claims and transmit a summary to the federal government. The government wrote the check, but whenever it wanted to audit bills, a pro-hospital intermediary stood between the government and the original paperwork in the hospitals. Furthermore, the rules on what were costs were vague and generous. They included money to amortize the expense of new equipment.

Physicians kept their cherished doctor-patient relationship, too. That is, they charged each individual patient a fee for service. Medicare

Part B reimbursed the doctor. There was no uniform rate schedule. The result was a bonanza for many physicians, not to mention plenty of outright fraud. In the mid-1970s the federal government began to combat these problems with regulations and inspections, but it did so only with difficulty and after the medical establishment had ballooned in size on a feast of federal money.

Federal Medicare spending went from $3.4 billion in fiscal year 1967 to $11.3 billion in 1974.[23]

Federal Government Health Outlays (percent of total)[24]

	1966	1970	1980	1990
Medicare	0.8	3.6	6.0	8.7
Medicaid	0.7	1.4	2.3	3.4
Health and hospitals	1.6	1.7	1.5	1.4
Veterans	0.9	1.0	1.1	1.1
Subtotal of medical items	3.9	7.7	11.0	14.6

Incidentally, the table shows that Medicaid, which is health care for the poor, grew considerably less than Medicare insurance for the aged. (The state governments also pay for Medicaid, but their share has increased more slowly than the federal portion.)

The annual rate of inflation for hospital bills was under 7% from 1950 to 1960. After Medicare came in, their charges rose at nearly 15% from March 1966 to March 1970.[25]

Feeding at the Trough: Insurance Companies

A growing market attracts profit-seekers. In the case of health care from the mid-1960s, the profit-seekers included insurance companies, hospitals both profit and non-profit, and new corporate forms of medicine.

Insurance companies began by undermining the virtual monopoly of Blue Cross. In school and in the newspaper, we are taught that monopoly is bad and competition is good, but in the corporate world things are not so simple. Blue Cross basically charged a uniform rate to all its clients in a region. Commercial insurance companies did not compete by offering a lower rate to everyone. Instead, they found ways to sign up only the people who brought the least risk of actually needing the medical service which is the end purpose of health insurance. Commercial insurers competed by aggressively soliciting the business of employers whose employees were young and better paid while responding lazily to people more likely to have health problems. Insurers charge higher premiums for groups and individuals judged to be greater risks, meaning that the persons most likely to need medical care are least likely to have coverage.[26]

We agree that someone who chooses to buy an expensive but fragile Corvette pays more to insure his automobile than does the owner of a plain Chevy. We live with the fact that young drivers pay more for insurance than middle-aged drivers. Most people, however, feel a moral dilemma if asked to accept that health care for a 50-year-old worker in a steel mill should cost him more and be less available than for a 25-year-old computer programmer. Skimming is a fundamental problem in any system of private health insurance; it is built into the competition for profits.

Feeding at the Trough: Hospitals

Hospitals have taken an increasing part of the expanding health care market.

Share of National Health Spending (percent)[27]

	1929	1940	1950	1960	1970	1980
Hospital care	18	25	30	34	37	40
Physicians	28	24	22	21	19	19
Drugs	17	16	14	14	11	8
Nursing homes	-	1	2	2	6	8
Dentists	13	11	8	7	6	6
Other	24	23	24	22	21	19

Some of the early expansion of hospitals follows from the growth of cities and related social changes. As individuals became more isolated in society, traditional places for convalescence and recuperation were no longer available. On the farm a family member might stay in bed. In a big city, a single individual in an apartment who needs nursing help is more likely to go to a hospital.

A big reason why hospitals pulled medicine into their premises is equipment and technology. A century ago a doctor could carry a stethoscope in his black bag to your house. Today he has someone look into you with equipment that puts out X-rays and magnetic fields. However, a doctor does not use each of these expensive machines every day. The hospital takes advantage of an economy of scale by having the machine available for a pool of physicians. The trend to the high-technology hospital site is a fact. However, it was not entirely a technical necessity, as we shall see later.

Medicare Part A allowed hospitals to include the cost of equipment in the bill and be reimbursed for it, but the federal government originally had little or no control over the decision to buy equipment. Hospitals had every incentive to get the latest machine. A study of open-heart surgery in California in 1976 found enormous duplication of the elaborate setups required to perform these operations. Ninety-one hospitals offered open-heart surgery, so most were idle most of the time. If there were only 30 centers, each performing one or two operations a day, the saving was calculated to be nearly one-fourth the total costs of such surgery.[28]

Along with simple growth since 1930, hospitals have taken new economic forms in the last 25 years. Chains of hospitals appeared. For one thing, they have easier access to debt markets. By 1980, 176 such corporations owned or managed 300,000 beds.

Between 1980 and 1991, almost 200 hospital mergers occurred.[29]

Investors took ownership of hospitals and ran them for profit. By 1970 there were 29 investor-owned, openly for-profit chains. Hospital Corporation of America controlled 23 hospitals in 1970; it grew to 300 in 1980, managing 43,000 beds. Today, the world's largest for-profit hospital company has annual revenue exceeding $10 billion; its co-founder, Richard Rainwater, got into the industry after serving as top financial lieutenant to the Bass family of Texas oil barons. The president of Humana, formed in Louisville, Kentucky in 1968, said he wanted to supply a product from coast to coast as predictable and reliable as the MacDonald's hamburger.[30]

At first sight, for-profit hospitals look like a small part of the scene.

Hospital Beds in 1980 (thousands)[31]

Nonprofit nongovernment	673
For-profit	87
State and local govt.	200

As of 1982, hospitals run for the purpose of generating profits had substantial market shares in a few states: California, Texas, Tennessee, and Florida. Health capitalists invade the most lucrative locations first. It is misleading, therefore, to average their presence over the entire U.S. Other parts of the country can see what heads their way by looking at the situation in vanguard California and among the retirees of south Florida, where Humana Medical Plan enrolled 54,000 people in 1991, but 33,000 quit.[32]

Although there is a legal distinction between profit and nonprofit, in a business society the term "nonprofit" is often deceptive, and the economic difference is small. Nonprofit hospitals set goals and act like for-profit companies. They both seek to expand, because a larger hospital has advantages in the competition for revenues. It can spread costs like advertising, the mortgage bonds on the buildings, equipment, and expensive salaries for the top executives over a larger number of patients. This advantage can be vital for survival during a downturn in business and helps a hospital to compete in general. The struggle is conducted between one hospital and another, and also between hospitals and managed care businesses that operate health centers of their own.

Hospitals and other medical corporations have become experts at mixing business units in favor of profit. For example, in the Bay Area east of San Francisco, most people know Alta Bates as a hospital. Old-timers might have heard that nurse Alta Alice Miner Bates started the medical center in 1905. Alta Bates went corporate in the late 1970s. It became a tangle of interests in partnerships, management contracts, profit corporations and formally nonprofit companies:

> Valley Care Imaging Associates, Valley Surgical Partners, Magnetic Imaging Affiliates, Alta CT Services, Alta Imaging Medical Group, Health Enterprises Facilities, Bay Mesh, Alta Bates Corporation, Alta Bates Medical Center, Guardian Foundation, East Bay Health Funding, Inc., California Healthcare System, Visiting Nurse Association & Hospice of Northern California, Visiting Nurse Association Private Care, Inc., Alta Bates Foundation, Alameda Hospital, Alta Bates Medical Resources, Alta Bates Medical Group, and Alta Bates Medical Associates.[33]

The boards of directors of these organizations overlap heavily. They steer revenues through the conglomeration by means of rigged prices that one unit charges another, loans made and later written off, and other mysterious ways. Money surges out of nonprofit hospitals, which bewail their condition, and into corporations and partnerships where a small circle of medical executives, investors, and physicians reap big returns.

Profit or nonprofit, hospitals are controlled by a privileged few. Patients as well as the bulk of the employees (orderlies, attendants, clerks, and most nurses) are definitely not part of the governing and benefiting group. The latter consists of many of the physicians associated with the hospital (except the residents), top administrators, insurance companies, prescription drug manufacturers, medical equipment vendors, and other suppliers. They all have their fingers in the pie.

Class Divisions: Physicians

The physician was the major economic player in hands-on medicine at the beginning of the century. Of 331,000 health care workers, making up 1% of the civilian labor force, one-third were physicians; about one-third were nurses, attendants and midwives; and the remaining third were veterinarians, pharmacists, dentists and lens makers and grinders.[34] It was the craft era of medical practice. Clerks, administrators, and various kinds of technicians were not in this picture.

In 1910 the M.D.'s issued the Flexner report, which made a sacred rule that the only legitimate and legal practitioner of medicine was someone who had a state license issued after he graduated from a medical school approved by an arm of the AMA. In the next decade it looked as though the AMA would go along with a proposal from a group of Progressive reformers for comprehensive health insurance. However, at its 1920 annual meeting the AMA fixed the course that it maintained until a few years ago: we doctors will accept clients one by one and charge them the fee that we decide is appropriate, and no one can start any insurance scheme, clinic, or government plan that we think is a menace to the way we do business. They even opposed the 1921 Sheppard-Towner Act, a mild federal law that put a little money into prenatal care and child welfare work, such as telling mothers about the need to buy unspoiled milk.[35]

In denouncing the Progressives' ideas for health insurance, physicians followed the lead of the commercial life insurance companies. In 1916, Prudential Insurance Company opposed health insurance because the Progressives had included funeral benefits, and insurance companies saw a threat to 44 million policies they had written.[36]

By 1930, doctors were down to one-fifth of the labor force in health care—the dominating elite within the medical world. Thereafter, as seen in a previous table, the physicians' share of the (growing) health care dollars declined from 1930 to 1950 to about 20%, but they still control another 60% of spending. Hospital administrators, for example, have a love-hate relation with physicians. Doctors associated with a hospital are by their referrals the source of business, but they assume they are lords of the manor, too. The magnates of for-profit hospitals solicit physicians as investors on the theory that they will send patients to them.[37]

By 1980, physicians were only one in twelve of health care workers.[38] Since then, their proportion has shrunk a little more. The ranks of technicians swelled and their work was divided into more specialties. During the 1980s, the number of people employed in health care increased rapidly (about 50% from 1980 to 1992). Enjoying the fastest growth over and above the expansion of the entire industry were managers, administrative personnel, and clerks. Nurses did not keep pace.[39]

Among physicians, more train to be specialists. The number of general practitioners per 100,000 Americans declined from 83 in 1940 to 32 in 1967. In only five years from 1965 to 1970, the percentage of doctors in general practice fell from 22% to 15%. The broader category of primary care providers, which counts pediatricians and general internists, too, is about one-third of practicing physicians, but in recent years only one-fourth of new doctors have gone into primary care.[40]

We all know that specialists make more money. In 1990 the median income for general family practitioners was $93,000; for a surgeon, it was $200,000.[41] The difference reflects the fact that medicine in the United States is *crisis medicine*. Car manufacturers spend millions of dollars persuading buyers to think that there are real differences between a Buick and Cadillac, for example. The situation for doctors works to the specialists' favor naturally. Simply let the condition become acute. The required treatment is more specific. When the patient needs a heart surgeon, a bone cutter won't do. Because preventive medicine and public health programs are starved of resources, the situation guarantees that many patients will develop a wide variety of problems, each requiring its own particular specialist who enjoys a seller's market at the moment of crisis.

The average income for doctors, excluding residents, in 1991 was $170,000. Between 1983 and 1990, their earnings rose 21% *after* inflation, while large numbers of working Americans fell behind inflation. [42]

Doctors are separating from each other in class terms, too. A few of them become entrepreneurs who launch clinics, preferred provider organizations, and other new forms of medical practice. A few more become top managers, helping large insurance and other corporations to enter the fray.

The ranks of doctors who neither employ more than an assistant nor are employed themselves are breaking up. The physician needs a closer tie to the expensive means of medical treatment housed in hospitals and elsewhere. He needs to be part of a marketing group, because everyone else is marketing. He needs more help with billing, collecting, and forms, which in a doctor's office typically take 40% of his gross revenue.[43] Already by 1981, one-fourth of physicians had formal contracts with hospitals, and three out of five of these were on salary. Physicians are also going on contract with managed care plans. Often the pay is generous, but for better and worse, doctors will slowly lose their autonomous position.

Fighting Corporate Attack: Health Care Workers

The term "cost control" means different things to different economic interests. Patients and ordinary citizens might hope that cost control would mean eliminating administrative waste, sales commissions and the excesses of marketing. To the executives of the health industry, however, cost control means reducing the wages of health care workers, laying them off and speeding up the remaining staff, breaking unions, and watering down the quality of medical service received by patients.

Wages fell from 56% of total hospital expense in 1972 to 44% in 1991. The cost of all grades of nurses fell from 23% of total expense in 1980 to 19% in 1990. Nursing assistants and the lowest-paid hospital service workers lost 13% to 16% of the buying power in their wages during the 1980s. The average base pay for full-time hospital service workers in 1991 was $14,000.[44]

Meanwhile, the average salary of a top administrator increased 50% in the 1981-91 decade to $90,000. Hospitals now have CEOs (chief executive officers) just like other corporations. The compensation paid CEOs of hospitals with 500 beds or more averaged $235,000 in 1992. Firms in the health care industry like American Practices Management, Inc., specialize in advising hospitals how to downsize, fire, lay off, and force retirement with minimum damage to public image, for a fee that typically runs to three-quarters of a million dollars.[45]

A survey of acute care nurses reported that 45% of hospital accidents result from inadequate staffing levels.[46]

Marin General Hospital in Greenbrae, California, converted in 1985 from public status to a private but still allegedly nonprofit board of directors. In July 1993, all 540 registered nurses lost their jobs. They were invited to bid against each other for a smaller number of jobs. At the same time, MGH denied nurses part-time and flex-time options they had enjoyed until then. As a result, many experienced senior nurses gave up their work in order to meet family responsibilities. The previous two years, the hospital reported profits of $5.6 million and $4.1 million.[47]

Alta Bates Corporation, a northern California medical conglomerate, spun off clinical laboratories into a new corporation, Pathology Institute. PI sold lab tests to the Medical Center at money-losing prices discounted 40% below market rates. After a few years the wheeler-dealers of Alta Bates exhausted the financial advantages of this scheme. They sold the outpatient accounts, folded the lab into the Medical Center, and used the corporate switch to repudiate the medical technicians' union contract. The technicians lost their union protection while a case brought by the National Labor Relations Board drags through the courts.[48]

Another bitter but this time successful conflict between executives and staff in corporatized medicine occurred at Summit Medical Center in Oakland, California, in the summer of 1992. The seeds of conflict grew from a typical bit of wheeling and dealing, the merger of several hospitals into Summit Medical Center. Summit executives demanded that five unions agree that none would honor picket lines set up by another of them. Some of the pre-merger hospitals had language for sympathy strikes, while other agreements were silent on the question. The workers refused to give up this right, saying that it was basic to the very principle of collective action.

On May 26, 1,700 hospital workers walked off the job and shut Summit down. Management spent millions to fight the strike. It brought in strikebreakers from out of state, paying them up to $50 per hour plus hotel lodging. Summit's top boss rejected compromises offered by union negotiators, and he refused terms worked out by a federal mediator with equal disdain. However, the workers held firm for six weeks. Jesse Jackson, Jerry Brown (then a candidate for President), and most East Bay politicians spoke at weekend rallies for the strikers. Although management did not concede the right to sympathy strikes plain and simple, the contract permits them if the workers are determined enough. In a sense, the issue was postponed, but Summit bosses were considerably weakened. Shortly afterwards, the chief executive officer left his post.

Technology Is Not the Answer

Technology has not reduced the cost of health care, and despite miracles in specific cases, new technology alone has not and cannot achieve good health care, especially economical, high quality care for large numbers of patients.

The United States is the undisputed leader in medical technology. Princes fly in from around the world to cure the results of living the rich life. Rock star and former world-class drinker David Crosby got a new liver. However, the U.S. population as a whole ranks below most developed nations in measures of health. Infant mortality is higher than in 20 other countries.[49] A man in the United States can expect to live a year less than a man in the United Kingdom.[50] (In today's political climate of blaming everything on immigrants, we must note that the U.K. has plenty of immigrants from its former colonies.)

Competitive duplication of high technology items reduces the quality of health care. California's overstock of heart surgery facilities means that the surgical teams in more than a third of them do not maintain their competence at top levels. The result is death rates as high as one patient out of six.[51]

The U.S. is overstocked with 10,000 mammography machines—five times as many as current demand justifies, and twice as many as full testing in an ideal world for all women requires. The price is higher because of the reduced volume of tests per machine, which has the result of turning a good thing into bad, since fewer women can afford the test.[52]

Eventually, giant health care corporations may reduce the duplication of equipment, but they will not break the cost spiral with new technology.

Instead, the fundamental condition for technology that improves health without raising costs is a change from crisis medicine to a system of public health. This means universal prevention (like inoculation), education, checkup for warning signs, and cheap mass testing (something that technology can help make possible). Public health programs have high volume—everyone, and they aim at early, simple conditions.

Crisis medicine is the opposite of public health. It waits for a problem to become severe. A variety of specialized, serious conditions generate demand for highly skilled specialists, elaborate machinery for treatment, and more time in the hospital. As we saw, crisis medicine creates a seller's market for the specialist physician as opposed to primary care doctors. It creates demand for high-profit operations sold by hospitals. Crisis medicine is practiced by a health system that is fragmented instead of universal, one whose time horizon is the corporate income statement rather than the lifetime of all citizens.

Corporatized Medicine

Health care has attracted corporate capital in the last two decades, and the trend is still young. The health crisis is a result of the corporate invasion and the changing relations between the different businessmen contending for revenue.

U. S. Corporate Profits After Taxes ($ millions)[53]

	1965	1970	1980	1990
All domestic corp.	41,874	34,770	117,945	227,063
Health services	47	218	2,190	5,010

Statistics on corporate profits recorded only a blip under the heading of health services in 1965. From then to 1990, corporations found money in health services at a pace almost 20 times greater than profits in general.

It is estimated that at least one-fourth of the money spent on medical care now goes to investor-owned companies.[54]

Among HMOs in California, the percent that are non-profit fell from 84% in 1980 to under 35% in 1994.[55]

Some of these corporations are insurance companies; some are new corporate oligarchs that insert themselves into the health care loop. The largest ones explore ways to combine insurance with the medical industry itself. The term "managed care" applies to a variety of ties between financial coverage and health work. From 1986 to the end of 1994, enrollment in managed care plans in all their forms increased from 26 million to 50 million people, of which 70% are enrolled in 266 plans owned by the ten largest firms. Counting HMOs exclusive of the looser preferred provider groups, they enroll one in five of all people in the U.S., and they are taking over one regional market after another.[56]

The managed care business may be a classic HMO, owning health centers and hiring doctors and other staff to work in them. Since 1970, however, the HMO label has been used more loosely. What is today called an HMO typically signs up physicians who continue to work in their offices. To an HMO, an important quality of a doctor is the hospitals at which he has admitting privileges. The HMO may pay the doctor a flat capitation fee per enrollee; the physician sees those enrollees who come in with a medical problem. Or the HMO may pay the doctor in the traditional manner of fee for service. Customers enroll with a managed care organization and receive what the HMO may call comprehensive care, or a defined set of coverages limited by exclusions, deductibles and copayments in the manner of typical health insurance policies.

The HMO label certainly lost the cooperative, socially-minded connotation that it had in the 1930s. When the Nixon administration offered legislation to encourage HMOs in 1973, *Fortune* magazine touted that their profit rate could match that of the oil companies.[57]

Nixon promoted HMOs as an alternative to a proposal that resembled what we call single payer insurance today. As Paul Ellwood, M.D., one of the thinkers behind the term wrote, "Most important, the health maintenance strategy offers a common cause for the collaboration of the professional, public, and private enterprise sectors of the health industry…as a feasible alternative to a nationalized health system."[58] In plain language, he said that doctors and corporate investors in the health business should get together and protect themselves from the threat of reform.

Today about 1,200 companies write health insurance. Most of them will be driven out of the field as the top five push managed care businesses requiring more capital than the small companies have.[59] The top five are Prudential, Cigna, Aetna, Travelers, and Metropolitan Life. (In mid-1994, the last two merged their health insurance operations.[60]) The first two are especially active in managed care. A conflict has developed between these oligarchs in waiting and lesser insurance companies. It was the latter whose trade group, the Health Insurance Association of America, ran television commercials attacking health care reform in the autumn of 1993.

The pie of health plan premiums divides as follows: 25%, the top five insurance corporations; 25%, the 70 Blue Cross/Blue Shield groups; 16%, HMO companies; 34%, other insurers.[61] These percentages are changing rapidly.

Insurance companies know that many people have a gut dislike of financiers in medicine, and the insurers often hide their ventures. When Aetna Life & Casualty began a chain of company-owned doctors' offices, it started a new brand name because, admitted a spokesperson, "people reacted more positively in surveys to HealthWays than the Aetna name."[62]

When corporations make investments, they direct them to ventures promising the highest rate of return. Nonprofit medical conglomerates do the same thing with their surpluses. As government regulations attempt to control costs in traditional acute-care hospitals, health care corporations break out activities into new businesses, leaving government to catch up with free-standing diagnostic sites, home delivery, and specialized outpatient surgical clinics. These facilities, having different equipment, capital and service profiles, escape per-procedure rules that govern cost control. Meanwhile, they market their variety of services. We might joke about the day when prenatal care will come in brands, just as colas are Pepsi or Coke, but that is going too far. Health industry marketers will likely aspire to the dignity of Lincoln versus Oldsmobile.

Crisis Point

Managed care businesses, financed by insurance companies and other sources of capital, have not solved the problems of a commercial market in health insurance. On the contrary, corporatized medicine is the source of the crisis. It is a crisis of less for more, of exploding costs combined with spreading insecurity about getting care when we need it.

As described earlier, increases in benefits were once a substitute for money wages, which have drifted down since the late 1960s. This phase has passed. Now employers refuse to pay the price of health care benefits, premiums whose rise outpaces general inflation year after year. In the mere seven years from 1987 to 1993, the proportion of big employers who provide health care for their retirees shrank from 57% to 35%.[63]

Chrysler Corp. reports that it spends more money on health benefits than on the steel it buys to make cars. The company says that in 1988 it spent $700 per car made in the U.S. on health care, while in Canada the cost was $223. More important, the Japanese automakers spent $246 per car in their home country on health benefits.[64] Chrysler and a number of other Fortune 500 companies demand changes because of the global disadvantage that the U.S. commercial health insurance system imposes on them.

Before insurance companies became involved in managed care, they had little control over costs and cost increases. As entrants into the market, they were forced to deal lightly with physicians and hospitals, who could boycott patients covered by an insurance company they did not like. More important, one company could obtain little competitive advantage. For example, if it devised a policy that encouraged lower costs, other insurers could write the same terms almost immediately. If an insurer invested time and resources bringing a hospital or physician into line on a cost matter, most of the gain would trickle away to all the other companies whose patients used the facility, too.

Cost Control: Whose Costs?

Managed care was supposed to enable the insurance company to reduce costs. The insurer or other corporate owner would bring business efficiency to medicine. However, it has not worked out that way.

The ultimate key to cost control is the opposite of crisis medicine, that is, preventive medicine. Complete and thorough inoculation campaigns are part of it. So is a saturation of care at early phases of typical problems, such as prenatal examinations instead of tragic and expensive premature births, and monitoring for problems known to begin at each stage of life.

Yet the motivation for a health maintenance organization to spend on preventive medicine is limited. It is true that many HMOs offer annual checkups, measles shots for children, and well-baby examinations. Even in this respect, their record is spotty. Immunization rates at HMOs range from 60 to 85% when they should be well over 90%.[65] HMOs might want to detect serious diseases a year or so before they become obvious, too, in order to avoid elaborate operations and treatments.

The basic fact, however, is that managed care is a thing of the market. Employers shop around for HMOs to offer their employees, and HMOs compete to take customers away from one another. At the same time, the HMOs calculate the expenses that an employee group with a certain age and occupation profile is likely to generate. Workers, for their part, often have an annual signup period during which they may change their HMO. Thorough and universal preventive care requires expense up front in return for a significant reduction in health problems over the years ahead. An HMO does not want to spend extra money today, knowing that much of the reward is years away and will spread into society as a whole. HMO businessmen find that broad preventive care does not pay off in their quarterly and annual bottom-line calculations.[66] In a market supplied and ruled by managed care businesses, socially beneficial cost control is structurally out of reach.

By competing for customers and encouraging turnover, corporate health plans generate new costs of treatment. Either data on a patient must be transferred, usually incompletely, or a doctor at the new plan will simply repeat tests. If the patient and a physician at the old plan had built up a relationship, the doctor at a new plan starts out all over again and incurs new costs by practicing more defensive medicine and probing to get the whole picture of the individual.

Corporatized medicine did not reduce costs during its first waves of growth. The very years of the 1980s during which millions of people were herded into managed care empires were also years during which the cost of health care exploded. A hundred years ago, big corporations replaced crowds of small companies on the basis of economies of scale and techniques for reducing production costs. This model does not describe the invasion of corporate capital into health care. If anything, corporatized medicine introduces new costs. Competition means battles to get customers, not a contest to maximize genuine care per dollar charged. Slick campaigns increase marketing costs. Duplication of equipment continues in many instances.

For awhile the tangled web of interests among health care providers ensnares and brakes the drive to cost control, too. Insurers press doctors to avoid unnecessary procedures, but physicians counter with disputes over who can judge what is necessary. The supposed beneficiary of health care, the patient, may even dare to speak up and insist on getting what is right. Forms and telephone calls fly back and forth. This expensive battle waged in the name of utilization review is cost control under corporatized medicine.

At a certain point, corporatized medical capital acquires enough weight in the health care industry to restructure it. We are now at the moment when the corporate health industry reduces its expenses in order to enlarge its profits. Dollar price rises may slow down, but physicians, health care workers, and patients suffer the burden.

For example, managed care organizations take the decision of when to provide care out of the hands of patient and doctor. The typical rule is that the patient sees a family doctor or other gatekeeper first. When not tainted by business motives, the idea is a good one. Recently, however, the Kaiser group raised the caseload of its primary care doctor to 2,000. The 15-minute doctor visit is becoming the seven-minute visit. For General Electric and its managed care suppliers, a gatekeeper professional was not cost effective enough. GE employees in Boston cannot even call their doctor to ask for an appointment. They must go through a GE reviewer (and assume that the reviewer is looking at a computer screen of the employee's care usage as they speak).[67]

When insurers and employers manage health care together, official data is a weapon in their hands for use against the worker. At Coors Co., most workers fill out a health history in return for a 5% reduction on their insurance copayment. Questions ask how they get along with in-laws and pry into sexual difficulties. Employee Richard Fletcher, Coors knew from its files, had mumps when he was eight, smoked 30 cigarettes a day, had a vasectomy when he was 24, and was embarrassed by smelly feet. Two weeks after Coors demoted Fletcher from office work to manual labor, and after his wife, Judy, found him one day sobbing on the floor, he died of a heart attack. She filed for survivor's benefits. Coors scanned its file on Fletcher, said he died of smoking, and avoided paying Mrs. Fletcher.[68]

As medicine goes corporate, events reflect the structural change. Physicians become uneasy about the loss of professional status. Hospitals and not-for-profit group health plans like Kaiser react to the corporate drive into medicine by pursuing their own conglomeration and downsizing. Management demands that nurses and other health care workers cut corners. They are asked to sacrifice pay and even accept reductions in their own health package on the altar of competitiveness—while the men in suits at the top award each other big raises for leading their hospital or HMO into the new era.

Multi-Tiered Medicine

Finally, corporate cost control means minimizing benefits delivered to members. Oh yes, someone can have any level of benefits that she wants, provided she is willing to pay. The result is that commercial health care is inevitably *multi-tiered medicine*.

The stratification of health care may be blatant. For example, the company quotes a higher rate to a prospective customer burdened by a "pre-existing condition," or simply denies coverage. This is an open declaration that the principle of commercial insurance, calculating and averaging risks, has corrupted health care. For each corporate player in health care, good business practice requires this approach, but the refusal to sell a policy on the excuse of a phrase like pre-existing condition testifies that the system of corporatized medicine has reached the point of crisis.

Multi-tiered medicine comes in more subtle forms. Health plans occupy market positions. The fancy plans advertise their distinctive luxuries in the world of modern medicine, like getting through the phone line to the appointment desk in less than half an hour. Health plans crowd into the more lucrative markets, such as the young family of professional workers in the suburb, or the truly wealthy among the retired. Then one or two plans rediscover the downscale part of the market, which they exploit with high prices for bad service, much like inner-city supermarkets.

The guaranteed loser when insurance companies sell a variety of plans is the consumer. One plan might cover many visits to the doctor's office but have high deductibles for the charges of a hospital stay. Another plan might be the reverse. This "choice" forces the prospective customer to gamble whether she will at some time in the future more likely need frequent office visits, perhaps for an allergy that is difficult to diagnose, or a week in the hospital for surgery. Certainly, she can get a policy that covers both situations, but the price is too high for most people.

Surveys of customer satisfaction report that managed care groups paying their doctors on the old fee for service model earn the best rating.[69] Naturally, the groups with the highest satisfaction can charge more. It's like Saks Fifth Avenue and Wal-Mart.

For these reasons, a health market dominated by corporations cannot give all of us economical, high quality care. The companies may cut their expenses by raising the pressure on health care workers and by selling nice words and delivering less to enrollees and patients. These, however, are tactics of commerce, not a social improvement.

Multi-tiered medicine and the moral atmosphere of health care approached as a business corrupt the motivation of well-paid members of the industry. In a letter to the *S.F. Bay Guardian*, a physician associated with Children's Hospital in Oakland, California, publicly declared his objection to an article for implying "that the ability of wealthier consumers to purchase a wide range of health care services is unjust. Isn't this simply another example of trying to reduce us all to the lowest common denominator? Why shouldn't we be allowed to choose additional options if we can afford them?"[70] Beverly Hills had an internist for every 566 persons in 1988; nearby Compton had one for every 19,422 people.[71] If the lowest common denominator is not tolerable for Beverly Hills, then there is social injustice in Compton.

After growing for decades, the number of people with commercial health insurance peaked in 1982 and has fallen steadily since.[72] Insecurity has spread throughout the American people. On any given day, 40 million people have no health coverage of any kind, private or public. Every year over a million more people lose their health benefits, even during a period of so-called economic recovery.[73] Another 60 million have coverage with so many limitations that a major illness would leave them in financial ruin. Many people do not realize that their insurance has annual or lifetime dollar caps and that an injury or disease can easily run up hospital bills exceeding the limit. Other people know their insecurity all too well; about one-third of employed workers in middle-income families told an opinion poll that they stay in a job they would prefer to leave just to keep health coverage.[74]

On one hand, uninsured and underinsured people fear the unpredictable possibility of an acute crisis. On the other hand, people worry about a problem they know is coming but for which they see no solution: the high probability of needing long term care in later years, for themselves or a family member for whom they are responsible.

When large numbers of people tackle the health crisis as a political problem, they can solve it. Many countries have health care systems more successful than ours. Next we look briefly at international experience.

3

A Glance at Other Countries

Health care is better in other countries than in the United States. Among the top 24 developed countries, the United States ranks 16th in life expectancy for women and 17th for men, and 21st in infant mortality. A Harris poll showed that the citizens of Canada, most of western Europe, the U.K. and Japan are more satisfied with their health care than Americans are. Other countries spend less of their national product on health industries, too, and physicians are happy to serve the community at more reasonable pay.[75]

Income Ratio of Doctor to Average Worker, 1987 [76]

U.S.	5.4 times
Germany	4.2
Canada	3.7
Japan	2.4
U.K.	2.4

Most other countries spend less because they guarantee care for all their people. They have removed or greatly restricted the profit motive in health insurance, or they simply never let a commercial market develop. "Voluntary insurance preceded public legislation in all European countries, but these insurance funds were tied to labor groups, political groups, religious groups—not to health care providers and commercial companies, as in America."[77] For as long as a century, largely in response to an independent, politically active labor movement, other countries have avoided our crisis in health care.

Germany

Kaiser Wilhelm I's chancellor of the empire, Otto Bismarck, introduced compulsory health insurance for German workers in the early 1880s. Adapting traditional sickness funds, the government required employers and employees to pay into them at specified rates. In return, the workers got some medical care and funeral benefits as well as disability insurance.[78] Health coverage was Bismarck's carrot in his carrot-and-stick policy against Germany's workers, who created the first mass socialist party. He had outlawed the party in 1878; the workers struggled to reverse the ban and succeeded in 1890.

The compulsory sickness funds remain the core of Germany's health system today. There are about 1,200 of them, organized on geographic, craft and other lines. They are nonprofit, nongovernment organizations and include 85% of Germans; government funds cover everyone else. Coverage is therefore universal, although the administration is complex because it is a historical relic. It is also comprehensive: all doctors' bills are paid in full, as are hospital stays for up to a year. Basic dentistry is free. Prescriptions are filled for a few pennies.

A half dozen or so associations of sickness funds bargain with the physicians, who belong to their own national group. The two sides negotiate a global cap on cost, and individual doctors are paid by fee for service. A notable feature of the German system is that specialists earn only a little more than primary care providers. Doctors who work for hospitals are on salary and do not see patients outside the institution. Half the hospitals are public, 37% nonprofit, and 13% for-profit. Administrative costs for the German system are 5% of total health expenditures, versus about 13% for the U.S.[79]

German doctors have high incomes, but the rest of the health workers are poorly paid—about 60% of the average German worker's earnings (versus 90% in the United States).[80]

Like other developed countries after World War II, Germany was subject to economic forces that tended to raise health care as a percentage of the national economy. In 1977 the federal Health Care Cost Containment Act introduced annually negotiated global budgets.[81]

Health care was not the principal demand of the workers' movement when Bismarck introduced one of the first comprehensive social welfare laws of the industrial era. Bismarck accepted a welfare measure in order to weaken sentiment for socialism. Nevertheless, all classes agreed to the reform, and it is clearly a political and moral standard that profit-making in the field of health care must be regulated. This standard is not unchangeable, and recently Chancellor Kohl insisted that Germans must live with reduced social benefits. Among these programs, however, health care is probably more secure than others.

Sweden

Sweden is worth a note. It did not achieve universal health insurance until 1955. Care is financed from general tax revenues rather than dedicated payroll taxes on employer and employee. Health facilities are set up in a graded series around a central hospital for a region: clinics, specialized operations, and nursing homes. Their staffs are on salary.

Sweden's notable contribution is a strong emphasis on public health for children. The people believe that steady work with children greatly reduces health problems throughout life. A School Health Service takes over from the Child Welfare Service when the child enters school. It carries out preventive public health programs for the students and educates them in good health habits.[82]

United Kingdom

Reactionaries who brand all health reforms as "socialized medicine" typically charge Britain with being a primary example of the alleged horror, so let us see how the U.K. came to its system of universal care and just how socialist it is.

An emperor's chancellor introduced health insurance for workers in Germany. In the U.K. a Liberal, David Lloyd George, pushed the National Insurance Act through in 1911. It applied to workers making less than two pounds per week and paid benefits toward the fees of general practitioners but not specialists or hospital bills. The Liberals were not a working-class party. A British historian described Lloyd George, a lawyer from Wales, as a man "with the authentic chapel eloquence and a complete absence of scruples."[83] In 1911 a million workers went on strike, and like Bismarck, Lloyd George used the health care issue as a carrot to deflect workers' discontent.[84]Although some legislation was passed in later years, for example, during the Great Depression, the next major event was a wartime measure taken in 1940. The Emergency Medical Service was set up to run all hospitals and medical services. War is a scourge that we have yet to conquer, but sometimes it produces public institutions that work very well. Perhaps even businessmen feel they must go along with the urgent requirements of national interest, and selfish individuals lie low because their usual activities are unpatriotic.

The wartime Service was so good that the British people decided to go further after World War II. In 1946 Parliament approved the National Health Service Act, and by 1948 the National Health Service began full operation. It took over all municipal and nonprofit hospitals.

General practitioners can sign up with the Service and in turn enroll clients up to a maximum number. Any patient and general practitioner may mutually agree to establish their doctor-patient relationship. The Service pays the physician a capitation fee per client on his roster. Patients with an ailment see their doctor, who acts as a gatekeeper to the specialists. The latter are hospital-based and on salary, although they may see private patients on their own. General tax revenues finance the NHS. The well-to-do are free to visit private doctors and go to private hospitals. Otherwise, the whole system is as much government-run as our fire departments.

When the Service began in 1948, a burst of pent-up demand overwhelmed it. These first days are the origin of stories about delays for eyeglasses and the like.

Is the National Health Service an example of socialism? Physicians accepted an income closer to the average worker's than under health insurance schemes in any other country. Hospitals were not run as expanding empires. However, the U.K. as a whole kept a capitalist economy, and inevitably a nationalized health service has connections to profit-making. For example, drug manufacture remained strictly a business, and Britain has several big companies like Glaxo, which sells one of the top-selling pharmaceutical drugs in the world, Zantac.

Health results appear to be good, although the life expectancy of women is low for a developed country—equal to the U.S. figure.[85] A National Health Service opens the door to giving public health top priority, but a political struggle is required to carry out prevention on a wide scale.

The U.K. spends about 6% of GNP on health care.[86] With the steady decline of the U.K.'s economic position in the world since World War II, health care has been constrained like other sectors of the economy.

A nationalized health system is an unsecured advance point. It comes under political attack and economic pressure, so the people who benefit must continually defend it. Business interests that want to grab the hospital industry keep pushing in. For example, they are allowed to bid for contracts to do hospital laundry and supply the food. This option becomes a club used to beat down wages of the hospital employees. Nevertheless, when President Reagan's political tutor, prime minister Margaret Thatcher, wanted to undermine the National Health Service in the 1980s, mass discontent forced the Conservative government to back off a good deal.

The NHS is not guaranteed a monopoly on providing health care. This feature might seem praiseworthy, because the sting of private competition should keep the NHS on its toes. However, private enterprise is not a necessity if a society wants to encourage competition. A socialist economy could set up NHS-A and NHS-B and let them strive to demonstrate which is more oriented to the public good and is more creative about realizing it. In the U.K., however, the competition is profit interests. Any failing of the NHS, in the absence of political defense by the citizens and rectification by public-minded staff, leaves an opening for private industry.

About one Briton out of four now has private health insurance.[87] This figure is an average, and the percentage is higher among more prosperous managers and professionals. It remains true that any citizen may use the National Health Service, but when care is not comprehensive and people feel compelled to buy their own policy, everyone is no longer in one boat. People at upper and upper-middle income levels resent having to contribute to the NHS. The service is in danger of becoming a resource-starved social orphan, serving as a last resort for the poor.

The National Health Service is an example of social welfare in a business economy. It is not a case of socialism, which characterizes a society as a whole rather than individual sectors of an economy.

Japan

Without describing the institutions of health care in Japan, we note that like all other developed countries except the United States, it has universal coverage. Some observers attribute the long lives of the Japanese people to their diet and centuries-old cultural traditions.

Life Expectancy in Japan (years)[88]

	1947	1990
Men	50	75.9
Women	53	81.9

Life expectancy is not a fixed thing, as the table shows. Its dramatic extension over four decades demonstrates that people can make institutional and economic changes for the better rather than give up in the face of tradition.

North Vietnam

Whatever one thinks of the Vietnamese government, and whatever the situation in Vietnam today, we must concede that during the war they achieved health care miracles. In 1954 the infant mortality rate was huge, 400 per 1000 births. The Vietnamese adopted a measure similar to China's "barefoot doctors," training large numbers of paramedics who carried out specific, important tasks of health care in mass drives. The rest of the time, they farmed alongside the other villagers. Despite the horrors of war, by 1970 the rate of infant mortality had been reduced to 23 per 1000 births—lower than the U.S. rate of 26 per 1000 at that time.[89] This accomplishment reminds us of Britain's Emergency Medical Service during World War II. Can we figure out how to unite people for the common good and make social advances in peacetime?

Canada

For decades prior to the 1970s, the Canadian health system looked like the one in the U.S. Doctors provided service for a fee. Canada is as much a free enterprise economy as the U.S. There was one sign that things might be different there. In one of the provinces (roughly equivalent to our states), Saskatchewan, a 1947 measure adopted a tax which, with general revenues, paid hospital bills but not doctor fees.[90] Commercial hospital insurance lost most of its market in one province.

During the 1950s and '60s, health care took an increasing share of the Canadian economy, parallel with the rise in the United States. Saskatchewan pioneered again in 1967, and by 1971 Canada had a working national health program. At around this time the U.S. committed itself more fully to Medicare with its bonanzas for the medical establishment, rejecting universal health insurance one more time. Since then, health costs have climbed only slowly in Canada, while they took off in the U.S. Health care now takes about 9% of Canada's economy but has swollen to 14% in the U.S. and is still rising.[91]A public nonprofit agency in each province runs the single payer system, observing national rules in order to receive federal block grants. Everyone is enrolled, with a very few exceptions. Patients and doctors retain their relationship of mutual free choice. The system does not assign a patient to a physician, nor does it confine anyone to a list of eligible doctors in the style of U.S. employer-sponsored plans. Copayments and deductibles for covered service are eliminated. Treatment includes all acute care by hospitals and doctors. Provinces vary in other areas of coverage. Most supply prescription drugs only for senior citizens; long term care is typically about two-thirds covered.[92]

Government bureaucracy is a favorite whipping boy of profit interests in the health care field, but they never talk about huge corporate bureaucracies. Blue Cross/Blue Shield of Massachusetts requires a staff of more than 6,600 for its two and half million clients in New England. The provincial agency in British Columbia serves over three million residents with 435 workers. In fact, the staff who handle universal health insurance for all of Canada's 25 million people is smaller than the bureaucracy at just this one Blue Cross/Blue Shield.

With only a single payer, doctors who maintain their own office spend far less on billing and other clerical outlays. In fact, their counterparts in the U.S. pay 2.3 times as much for these costs. The Canadian advantage arises out of two differences. First, they submit one form to one payer, the provincial agency. More important, Canadian doctors do not fight bureaucratic wars with case reviewers, who are a standard operating tool of commercial insurers and managed care companies in the U.S.

Insurance overhead per person in Canada is $34; in the U.S. it is $212. As for paper-pushing in the facilities where health care is actually delivered, Canadian hospitals spend 9% of their budget on billing administration; U.S. hospitals spend 20%. If the United States reduced administrative costs to Canadian levels, besides saving $43 billion in direct insurance overhead, the country would save an even greater $49 billion on the administrative costs of hospital care, as well as $24 billion for such costs built into physicians' charges.[93]

Half the physicians in Canada are family doctors, while three-fourths of new U.S. physicians become specialists.[94] A patient is supposed to visit a specialist only when the family doctor refers her. This part of the system does not always work to control costs. A general practitioner who could treat a slightly complicated ailment may be happy to refer instead. He can see more patients and collect more fees while he generates goodwill among the specialists, too. A single payer setup attacks the main problem in health care today, commercial insurance, but it does not automatically cure all defects.

What are the results? Life expectancy in Canada is over a year and half longer than in the U.S. The U.S. Harris poll organization reported in 1989 on the results of asking Canadians and Americans about their health care systems. Have you had difficulty in getting needed treatment? With their universal insurance, Canadians almost never said they had difficulty for financial reasons, while 7% of Americans reported that they had found no safety net. Apart from lack of money, the poll asked whether other problems, such as long waits for operations or the absence of facilities in the area, had caused difficulty in getting needed care. Americans cited problems at twice the rate voiced by Canadians. A Canadian pollster says, "More than 90% of Canadians favor our system."[95]

Occasionally, a U.S. commentator alleges that Canadians suffer long waits for operations. This is not true. For example, more women in Washington state who are diagnosed with breast cancer wait at least three months for surgery than do women in neighboring British Columbia.[96] When the General Accounting Office of the U.S. government studied the Canadian system, it found no waiting in emergencies, short delays for urgent care, and longer waiting for elective care.[97] In the U.S., there is no waiting for those who have Cadillac health insurance, some waiting for other insured people, and disastrous waiting until the patient rolls into the emergency room for uninsured people.

Even where statistics show a wait, it helps to investigate how things really work. Some people want to visit a particular specialist. If she is popular enough to be a health care "star," we may concede that under the Canadian system her work hours still have only 60 minutes each. Also, physicians will add a patient to a waiting list before they know that the person really needs the operation. This practice reassures the patient that things are in motion, and it keeps both of them to a schedule for refining the diagnosis and making a firm decision about surgery.

U.S. opponents of the Canadian system concede in effect that perhaps 99% of the medicine there is passable, but Canadians must cross the border to our country for high technology operations. However, the numbers show that Canadians have comparable rates of showcase transplant surgery.

High-tech Transplants (per 100,000 people) [98]

	U.S.	Canada
Heart or lung	8.0	7.1
Kidney	39.4	31.9
Liver	6.8	7.5
Bone marrow	0.75	0.91

We should examine these figures and wonder instead how many unnecessary procedures are done, especially in the U.S.

Canada is not more of a welfare state than the U.S. Let us add private spending on health to all taxes, since in effect commercial insurers in the U.S. operate as payroll tax collectors. The result in 1990 was that both countries spend about 37% of gross domestic product on the combined sum of all taxation and health expenditures.[99]

Mass media in the U.S. give much play to charges that the Canadian health care is worse than the system here. In Nov. 1991 the *New York Times* said that women in Canada "must wait months for a simple Pap smear."[100] This statement is false, plain and simple, as the Canadian ambassador to the U.S. wrote to the *Times*.[101] Just as in the U.S., the woman's primary care doctor takes the Pap smear.

Polls by the *Los Angeles Times*, the Harris organization, and even the Health Insurance Association of America all report that 60% or more of people here in the U.S. prefer a Canadian-style system.[102] Ordinary Americans who have seen it in operation testify in its favor. Every now and then a letter to the editor gets into print. This one made it into the *San Francisco Chronicle*:

> During November 1992, I spent some time in Vancouver, British Columbia, on business. I asked about 35 Canadians what they thought of their medical system. They all gave their medical system high marks.
>
> A lady from Montreal has been in a wheelchair all her life and loves the system. Another person who was in a horrible automobile accident and told of his many operations can't say enough about the system.
>
> Another lady's father was visiting from the States, and had a very bad heart attack. He was in intensive care for over a week and the total bill was $40—for the ambulance that picked him up within five minutes. Others talked about the normal sicknesses they and their families had, and they all spoke very highly of their medical system.
>
> The people who use the medical system like it.
>
> I'm tired of listening to people in our government or people in authority in our medical system telling me how the Canadian medical system doesn't work. All I did was ask the people who use it and they love it and it gives them all peace of mind.
>
> —Todd H. Morrison, Redwood City[103]

In August 1994 the mayor and city council of Buffalo, New York, blocked out a "chain fast" on the calendar. Each official took one day and did not eat as a way of demanding that the U.S. adopt a single payer system. The city has a problem because with the decline of its heavy industries, workers who lost their jobs and their health coverage overwhelm the general hospital. The city knows about the single payer solution because it is only a ten-minute drive from Canada.

Twenty years ago Canada and the United States had similar health insurance systems. They faced the same financial problems. Then the Canadians went down a different path. Today, without spawning a big bureaucracy, they have universal coverage of all residents, comprehensive health service, and security (peace of mind, as Mr. Morrison wrote). Although the Canadian economy has its problems, a dollar-eating health care sector is not one of them. Americans, on the other hand, getting care only with the permission of a commercial insurance bureaucracy, are insecure about their health care. The health sector is one-seventh of the U.S. economy and still expanding.

Two questions that naturally arise are, why does the Canadian system work, and can Americans do the same or better? The answer to why is essentially that the Canadians do not depend on commercial health insurance. They decided that for this social function, a marketplace is not suitable.

As a consequence of their fundamental decision against commercial health insurance, Canadians reduced administrative costs. They avoided the expense and embarrassment of billboards and all the other apparatus of marketing health care like an automobile. They eliminated the financial hurdle to seeing a doctor when someone needs to see one, thereby promoting early treatment and improving health. They spared their economy the cost of duplicated high-tech facilities.

Those in the U.S. who deny the value of Canadian-style health care went through three phases of argument. At first, they told alarmist falsehoods, such as the myth about Pap smears noted above. Next, opponents of single payer care offered anecdotes that were outmatched ten to one and statistics that only revealed their artful misuse of figures. Also, they grabbed complaints by Canadians out of context. It is easy to do this, because as a public agency, Canada's health services get more citizen review than the lords of U.S. commercial insurance would ever stand for. However, Canadians are united on not wanting the mess that exists in the U.S.

In their third phase of denying the undeniable, the masters of debate simply dismissed Canadian experience as irrelevant because Canada is, they say, such a different society. Actually, no two major economies in the world are both more alike and more closely entwined with each other than the U.S. and Canada. Canada has ethnic divisions and immigrant minorities, too, like the French Canadians of Quebec and the Asian influx into Vancouver. Perhaps the U.S. commentators hint at one major difference: no industrial country on earth matches the U.S. when it comes to the intensity of racism. The problem with this allusion, however, is that health care run by the insurance companies has given tens of millions of people of every color insecurity and worry and high cost. More than any sermon by Martin Luther King, Jr., the barons of the health industry have taught Black, brown, yellow and white that we are all in this thing together.

4

Health Reform Fails in Washington, D.C.

Reform of health insurance took over the nation's agenda on Nov. 5, 1991. In a special election held to choose a senator from Pennsylvania, long shot Harris Wofford defeated former Attorney General Richard Thornburgh. Wofford built his campaign on the need to guarantee health security for everyone.[104]

Several presidential candidates in 1992 took up the issue of health reform, first Bob Kerrey then Bill Clinton. By the end of 1993 it appeared that something would be done. Among the alternatives in Congress was a single payer Canadian-style plan, sponsored by Rep. Jim McDermott (Dem.-Wash.) and 92 members of Congress. President Clinton eventually produced elaborate legislation, which he called managed competition. Moderate and conservative factions offered bills that would tinker with the health insurance market.

Campaign Promises

The Clinton campaign and presidency issued changing statements and proposals for health insurance. Two fundamental elements determined the substance of his position and the changes in it. One is that no plan from Clinton will deprive commercial insurance companies of their market and their profits made on health insurance and managed care ventures. The second requirement is that Clinton wanted to introduce some reform like universal coverage for which he could take credit by 1996.

In the summer of the 1992 election year, Clinton asked everyone to read his campaign document, *Putting People First*. The introductory summary committed his presidency to "providing quality, affordable health care by radically controlling costs, reducing paperwork, phasing in universal access to basic medical coverage, and cracking down on drug manufacturers and insurance companies."

This campaign literature was the farthest that Clinton went toward reform. He joined the criticism of the current system, saying that it "does not work" and does not give us "our money's worth." He admitted the shame that "infants die at rates that exceed countries blessed with far fewer resources." He declared that insurance companies routinely deny coverage to consumers with pre-existing conditions, and he cited the hundreds of billions of dollars spent on health care, rising rapidly over the preceding twelve years. "Almost 60 million Americans have inadequate insurance—or none at all," he said. We "live in fear." He struck a class note: "Every year working men and women are forced to pay more while their employers cover less."

The candidate promised reforms. Count on him to be "cracking down on drug and insurance company practices" and to "stand up to the powerful insurance lobby." He would put national spending caps on the health care sector of the economy. He promised universal coverage and equal premiums for everyone in a community.

Putting People First had the rhetoric of major reform, but it also signaled the big insurance and managed care corporations that they had nothing serious to worry about. In fact, the new setup could help them at the expense of smaller players in the insurance and health care industries.

Clinton let watchful observers know that he would continue multi-tier coverage. This point is important to insurers so they can develop second-rate operations into which they herd the poor, the working poor and a good many middle-income families. Meanwhile, the insurers sell grades of more acceptable coverage at a higher premium. The government cannot buy everyone a Cadillac; people who want adequate medical care will pay extra.

Therefore, candidate Clinton pledged to phase in "universal access to basic medical coverage." He spoke of a "core benefits package." At the time, he included prescription drugs for all, as well as some mental health and long term care. The specific items do not matter much. By repeating words like "basic" and "core," Clinton established his point that a multi-tier system would remain.

Close readers of Clinton's pitch (and everyone should be a careful observer of this man who in Arkansas earned the name "slick Willie") also found that he ruled out the single payer option in advance. Instead, "companies will be required to insure their employees...." Or, at least, "employers and employees will either purchase private insurance or opt to buy into a high quality public program." Commercial insurance corporations knew that they would continue to be the sellers in a lucrative market.

Clinton also had enough advice from the policy whizzes of the insurance industry that he could specifically endorse "managed care networks" that "will receive a fixed amount of money for each consumer...." Big HMO chains knew they had their man.

Taking on the insurance industry turned out to mean, "We need to streamline the industry. My health plan will institute a single claim form" and tell every insurer "to take all comers...[at] the same rate." The idea of one claim form for hospitals dealing with multiple insurance corporations is a cheap parody of cutting administrative costs. Administrative expense is an issue of how the health care industry is organized, much more than a matter of standardizing a form.

Insurance companies live by avoiding high-risk and high-cost enrollees and by charging more and delivering less in accordance with risk. The essence of competition between insurers is playing this game. It is good to have a rule against openly denying coverage for pre-existing conditions. It is another and near-impossible task to keep profit-seeking insurers from skewing their client populations. Companies locate their best facilities in one part of town and under-staffed clinics in poorer neighborhoods. They steer unknowing enrollees to one doctor or another in the plan, market aggressively to desired groups and provide signup information to other people only when they firmly request it. An existing regulatory system, Medicaid, has found it impossible to win the cat and mouse game of chasing after insurance corporations that know where they want to do business and where they do not. But Clinton pressed on.

One more point about *Putting People First* is its attack on prescription drug firms. It is true that the rate of return on capital in the pharmaceutical companies is at the top of the list of all corporations.

Clinton criticized the drug and insurance companies together several times, sometimes mentioning one first, sometimes the other. However, the share of national health spending going toward prescription drugs has fallen by half in the last 30 years to well under 10%.[105] The key players are the health insurers. (As we will see, a single payer attack on the insurance corporations would pay an extra dividend by means of pooled buying power for drugs.) By pairing the two villains, Clinton reduced his attack on the insurers to specific odious practices, playing down their large and growing power in the health business as a whole.

Health Alliances

After winning the election, President Clinton set up a health care task force. Hillary Clinton was its chief executive, and management consultant Ira Magaziner was the chief operating officer. The policy group put the two elements of the Clinton position—protect the big commercial insurance and managed care corporations, but reform something—into a different relation with each other.

The key to reform became an intricate organization placed on top of the existing setup. States and regions would form health alliances. Most employers and employees would be required by law to join the alliance and purchase insurance through it. This body in turn would negotiate with insurance and managed care corporations like Cigna, then retail the policies to its members.

Alliances would offer three health policies, perhaps more in some places. One would be an HMO that would provide the core benefit package. Another would let you go to doctors who charge a fee for service. The third was a blend of the two basic types. There would be deductibles and copayments. In other words, multi-tier medicine is alive and well.

Clinton introduced the handiwork of the task force with a major speech on Sept. 22, 1993. This was his rhetorical high-water mark. He earned praise for a moving, noble presentation emphasizing values rather than details. He laid out six principles for health care: "Security, simplicity, savings, choice, quality and responsibility."[106]He promised coverage "comparable to the benefit package offered by most Fortune

500 companies." Cost caps were essential, including government ceilings on price increases. Clinton still talked about one standard insurance form as a magic weapon, although now he gave equal emphasis to a need to "simplify the government's rules and regulations…" (at the same time that the health alliances would keep insurers to the straight and narrow).

Except for a jab against denying coverage to people with preexisting conditions, Clinton no longer bashed the insurance corporations. He turned to criticizing, ever so gently, the mass of the people. "Many of us…have used the system whether we needed it or not…" Apparently, we must have a greater sense of responsibility than to enjoy hanging out in the waiting room at the clinic when nothing is wrong with us.

The September 1993 speech and the first leak of details from a massive piece of legislation were only holding actions. Congress would not take up health care until 1994. The subject dropped off the nightly news. In the business press and in Washington, the health alliances came under attack as a fragile and unworkable tangle. Also, critics noted that Clinton's numbers were fantasy: he could not pay for the reform measures he wanted. On Feb. 8, 1994, the Congressional Budget Office confirmed that Clinton's plan would not save money but would instead require an infusion of funds. Business executives in health care decided that they did not like the price controls.

The Clinton plan was terminally ill. The question of the day shifted down to what kind of compromise reform might be legislated.

From Tug of War to Mutual Collapse

Every special interest in the health industry—big insurance companies and middle-sized ones, the managed care industry, employers who provide health benefits and those that do not, big corporations and small business, hospitals, and physicians—rolled into Washington, D.C., with fat bankrolls and slick lobbyists. In the end, and in the absence of any leader concerned either with the general welfare or even the broadest interest of the business class as a whole, the result nearly a year later was nothing. It was like a tug of war that ends with both sides collapsing to the ground at the same time.

Between September 1993 and February 1994, one political clash flared. The Health Insurance Association of America spent fourteen million dollars on television commercials. "Harry and Louise" sitting at the kitchen table discuss a problem with the Clinton plan and conclude with a sigh that there must be a better way (which their script carefully avoids). Hillary Clinton gave a speech in reply, working herself up to demand of the insurance companies, "We want our health care system back." The HIAA brings together about 300 medium-size companies in the industry. In the event that the government promotes managed care organizations, the top five insurers will prosper, while HIAA member companies, which mostly push paper and lack the resources to run HMOs, will have to leave the market. Ms. Clinton is a champion of the biggest insurers. She used a fight with the smaller companies of the HIAA to posture as little David fighting for the people.

> "For [Prudential] the best-case scenario for reform—preferable even to the status quo—would be enactment of a managed competition proposal."—Bill Link, executive vice president, Prudential Insurance Company.[107]

Clinton returned to health care reform in his state of the union address on Jan. 25, 1994. Now he needed to pull all the special interests together for a piece of legislation. The relation between the desire to stamp his name on a reform law and his basic acceptance of commercial health insurance changed again. His speech laid these two elements side by side in irrational contrast. On one hand, Clinton said, "In today's health care system, insurance companies call the shots. They pick whom they cover and how they cover them. They can cut off your benefits when you need your coverage the most. They are in charge."

Just three paragraphs later, Clinton showed they were in charge of him. He praised "what works today in the private sector...employer-based coverage" and carefully promised "private insurance for every American."

"And I might say, employer-based private insurance for every American was proposed 20 years ago by President Richard Nixon to the United States Congress. It was a good idea then, and it's a better idea today." Nixon and Clinton both took the advice of Paul Ellwood,

M.D., the man who promoted HMOs to avoid national health insurance, the man who convened top insurance executives at his home in Jackson Hole, Wyoming, and hammered out strategies to increase their dominance of health care.

Insurance companies, according to the President, must enjoy the duty of having to sell their product to every American. This is their brand of universal coverage. Naturally, they are in business to make a profit. Your choice is loophole-ridden benefits that you can afford or complete treatment that only high-income persons can buy.

Clinton also moved toward legislation by undercutting the elaborate apparatus of health alliances that were dear to the policy designers in his task force. He said he was open to the best ideas from any party. He insisted only on private health insurance for every American—universal coverage it must be, but comprehensive and sufficient in the basic package it need not be. Clinton would sign any bill, threatening only to veto anything that he could not label, however lamely, universal.

Within a week and a half of the state of the union address, both the Business Roundtable, a group of Fortune 500 top executives, and the U.S. Chamber of Commerce, which reaches down to middle-sized corporations, came out against the Clinton task force's proposals.

A Tennessee congressman named Jim Cooper began to get publicity for his proposals in place of the Clinton scheme. This occurred while, in the period from July to December 1993, fully 30% of Cooper's large-donor money came from health interests.[108] He suggested tax incentives to help people buy health insurance (which are worth more to upper-income people in higher tax brackets than to lower-income families). He tossed aside Clinton's health alliances and substituted modest government aid to help small businesses gather into buying cooperatives.[109]

At one point the Business Roundtable voted 60 to 20 to support Cooper's bill. But a writer from the Cato Institute, a right-wing group speaking for reactionary medium-size businesses, dubbed the plan Clinton Lite. He felt that Cooper's incentives would hasten the concentration of health insurers and health providers into managed care groups.[110]

Three Causes of Gridlock

Cooper's bill never got far. In this respect it foretold the outcome of every legislative effort for the rest of 1994. There were three basic reasons for this pattern. First, business sectors fought each other to a draw. What one special interest wanted was a negative for another. For example, some big corporations that provide health benefits, like Bethlehem Steel and American Airlines, wanted reform in order to control the rapidly increasing costs of those benefits. However, their proposals required that other companies pay more, such as fast-food chains and other employers that do not provide benefits. Small businesses that do not provide health policies now demanded, through the National Federation of Independent Businesses, tax subsidies for any mandate to provide coverage. For awhile, legislators played a bidding game with each other of writing larger subsidies, until big business objected.

So sharp and selfish was the war of business interests that it almost tore apart the U.S. Chamber of Commerce. Large companies in it wanted some kind of employer mandate because when small employers do not buy insurance, the insurers and hospitals engage in what is called "cost shifting," using higher premiums to cover services to the uninsured, usually provided in emergency rooms. Even though a proposed mandate was extremely weak (the employer would have to pay only 50% of the lowest-priced plan, a rule to be phased in only by the year 2000), small business members of the Chamber screamed no. The Indiana state Chamber of Commerce virtually seceded from the national organization.[111]

The second reason for the failure of proposals was the dilemma of coverage versus cost. As long as the commercial insurance companies run the health industry, taking their cut and injecting administrative expenses into their own operations as well as those of hospitals and other providers, the two goals of providing care for everyone and braking costs are mutually contradictory. For example, House leaders put forward a liberal plan seeking universal coverage through a mandate that employers must provide health benefits. In the existing structure of health care, such a mandate is inevitably costly. IBM executives got on the company's internal E-mail system and urged 180,000 U.S. employees to send objections to their representatives.[112] Other proposals dealt with cost but did not reach universal coverage. Every legislator faced the choice of either supporting a good amount of reform and finding money to pay for it, or merely tinkering with the health insurance market.

As 1994 wore on, strange words crept into news reports about the Washington debate, terms like "soft trigger vs. hard trigger." Week after week the scope of health reform narrowed. The call for universal care was reduced to a trivial debate over 85% versus 93%, in 1999 or at the turn of the century. Meanwhile, benefits shriveled so that at best they might give 100% of the people their own first aid kit (a suggestion that finally appeared in a lampoon on the television show *Saturday Night Live*).

Change in the health industry was the third reason why reform failed in Washington. As managed care corporations increased their dominance of the industry, they provided some price relief to big employers. Chrysler, originally an advocate of reform and cosponsor with American Airlines of a pro-Clinton coalition, lost enthusiasm when it realized what had happened. "A majority of Chrysler employees are now in managed care," said Walter Maher, director of federal relations for the automaker.[113] The big client corporations did not care that the change was at the expense of patients, health care workers, and people outside the markets served by managed care groups, as long as bills to the corporations stopped rising so rapidly. *Business Week* editorialized in a plea for enough reform to deal with cost shifting, "The mandated coverage could be bare-bones,..." as it praised the dramatic payoff of managed care to help big business "lower medical bills and monitor spending."[114]

The fate of Senator Wofford was a personal mirror of the fate of health reform. With nothing to show for his 1991 campaign theme of health care, and reducing himself to modest hopeful talk instead of a smashing call for basic change, Wofford lost his 1994 re-election bid.

Where was the single payer idea in all of this futile effort to make sausage (legislate)? The one position that the business sector of society could express as a general view was opposition to the single payer reform. This does not mean that, in a brand new debate, all of business would oppose single payer. Rather, insurance companies and many employers oppose it and were able to deny it national visibility. They set the establishment view from their position of dominance. It became irrelevant that the largest bloc of legislators sponsoring one measure was the 92 members who signed on to Rep. McDermott's single payer bill.

It must be admitted that some sponsors backed single payer in order to obtain bargaining leverage. For example, California's Ron Dellums wrote to his constituents in April 1994, "I will continue to push for this 'Canadian' model in the hopes of securing a better package."[115] Senator Wellstone, whose name was originally hyphenated with that of McDermott on the bill, drifted away from the group.

Lacking a prominent champion in the White House or elsewhere on the national scene, the single payer plan got almost no exposure from the corporate mass media. What was needed was a mass movement for single payer.

5

Californians Write a Single Payer Plan

When health care reform climbed to the top of the national agenda, Californians in favor of a single payer plan decided to do more than watch Congress and the President. In January 1994 they launched a petition drive in the state. Within 100 days they collected over one million signatures, enough to put the California Health Security Act on the November 8, 1994 ballot. It became Proposition 186.

Basic Idea of Single Payer Reform

Under the Health Security Act, every California resident receives a health security card that guarantees her right to care. She keeps her card regardless of how her job or marriage situation changes. Children, students, employed and unemployed, retired—everyone is covered.

A patient goes to any doctor or joins any health group. Doctors and hospitals treat her, take an imprint of her card, and are reimbursed by the single payer fund; she never sees a bill. If she needs tests, they are covered. If she is expecting a child, she gets prenatal care. If she should receive dialysis, she gets it. Treatment for substance abuse and mental illness is provided. Long term care is covered, preferably in her home, in an institution if required. There is one copayment: $5 for a prescription filled outside a hospital or doctor's office, waived for someone unable to pay.

Today, commercial insurers whittle away the benefits in any policy whose premium is affordable, drive upper middle income people to pay more for comprehensive treatment, and leave the rest of us with partial care. When a single payer replaces commercial insurers, their dance of market positioning ends. Medicine becomes high quality for everyone.

The doctor, hospital, or other provider bills the health security fund. Every patient's card is as good as anyone else's, and each patient can go to any doctor. The providers do not compete for individual patients on price but rather on quality. If the care is not good, the patient will go to someone else.

Consumer choice is total. Because the insurance is a right enjoyed by everyone instead of a privilege granted by your employer, he does not specify one or two managed care groups from whose staff you must choose. You go to any doctor's office or join any health plan registered with the public system.

Instead of purchasing a commercial insurance policy, with its premiums, deductibles, copayments, and annual and lifetime limits, California residents pay into a single payer fund. The rate is 2.5% of taxable income. For someone with a taxable income of $30,000, the amount works out to $63 a month. At low incomes, the payment is $50 per year for a household. As we will see, most of the money for the fund comes from existing government health spending and from a payroll tax replacing employers' outlays on benefits for their staff.

Every resident is covered regardless of her circumstances. She pays according to her ability in the form of a small income tax. There are no premiums, no rates determined by age, sex, and number of dependents. She does not get a bill and then get reimbursement for it; she simply presents her health security card.

By eliminating commercial insurance companies, the single payer fund can give every resident comprehensive health care as a right. Insurance companies spend 27 cents of every health care dollar on paperwork, advertising, marketing, sales commissions, profits, and big salaries for top executives. The health security fund spends no more than four cents on administration and at least 96 cents of every dollar on care.

Can We Give Away Health Care?

It promotes health when someone who feels something wrong has her condition checked without first worrying about a money barrier. Financial worry leads uninsured people to live with small problems until a crisis drives them into the emergency room, which is society's most costly setting for treatment. On the other hand, the ideology of promoting individual responsibility argues in favor of copayments and deductibles. Conservatives, economists, and New Democrats—all of them well-paid spokesmen for big capital who have no worries about their own care—say that people must be made aware of the cost of health treatment, or they will overuse an apparently free good. This argument applies to commodities like beer, telephone service, and maybe even toilet paper. It does not hold true for health care.

For a couple of years after a single payer plan goes into effect, a surge of existing complaints would wash through the system, judging by what happened when the National Health Service in the United Kingdom introduced universal care (in a different form than single payer insurance, which leaves actual care in the hands of private business). The rate of usage by low-income people would probably increase permanently, because they currently do not receive the care they need.

Without an up-front money barrier for the sick individual, the plan encourages her to get early treatment and preventive measures. Prenatal care, annual checkups, and the like under one universal system pay for themselves by reducing emergency room usage and by curing ailments with simple treatments before they develop to an advanced stage.

For example, by reaching out to mothers-to-be about prenatal checkups and guidance, the single payer fund avoids most of the intensive care required by seriously premature babies. Every dollar budgeted for prenatal care saves over three dollars in the cost of taking care of babies born with low birth-weight. The single payer plan, by issuing everyone a health security card, and knowing that residents today will in most cases be here in the years ahead, contains the economic incentive to promote prenatal, well-child and other forms of preventive care and early treatment. Private insurers, even HMOs, are oriented to their annual profit rate; they cannot make the long term approach to health care for everyone an economic reality.

Today it is not the insured patient who soaks up medical treatment without regard to cost. Instead, health providers generate activity not required for the purpose of doing health work. Twisted incentives guide physicians and hospitals. They see well-insured persons more than necessary in order to make up for what they count as losses taken to treat under-insured patients. On one hand, doctors pile on tests and order unnecessary procedures when they think they can get away with them, practicing defensive medicine. On the other hand, a physician skimps on treatment so that insurance companies and managed care bosses see him as a cost-effective practitioner.

The single payer plan does away with these results of multi-tiered, crisis medicine. The citizenry as a whole and their health commissioner can finally spend properly on public health and preventive care in order to save a lot in the medium and long term. After all, Canadians enjoy better health (longer life expectancy and lower infant mortality) and a lower bill for health care as a percent of their economy (9% of gross domestic product instead of more than 14%).

The California Health Security Act

The vision of single payer reform just described did not become reality on Nov. 8, 1994. Most voters knew very little about how the Act would work. Since future struggles begin where California's 1994 effort left off, we give a more detailed explanation of Proposition 186.

A group of doctors, health reform activists, and attorneys who had experience dealing with insurance companies wrote the Act. Although they took Canada's single payer system as a guide, they wrote tougher cost controls, and they decided to cap health spending at its existing portion of the California economy, about 14%.

In the rest of this chapter we examine details of the Act, quoting typical clauses and dealing with a few controversies along the way. It occupied 16 pages in the voters' pamphlet and takes 85 pages in a comfortable type size. Although it is long for a referendum item, Proposition 186 is succinct compared to the bills of 1500 pages and more that went nowhere in Congress.

Section 1 declares: "This initiative establishes a California health security system that will protect California consumers, taxpayers, and employers from the skyrocketing cost of health care. Savings will be achieved by limiting health care costs, eliminating waste, and emphasizing disease prevention. Under the time-tested single-payer system established by this act and administered by an elected Health

Commissioner, the practice of medicine will remain private. Under the health security system, all Californians will have free choice of health care provider, regardless of employment, and access to comprehensive health care, including long-term care. The health security system will provide these services for the same or less money in real dollars than is spent on health care in California today."

The "time-tested system" is Canada. Although the paragraph emphasizes cost saving, it declares in effect that health care is a right. Savings come from three sources. The main one is "eliminating waste," a bland way of announcing that the single payer plan is health care without insurance companies. We will reduce administration and other non-medical expenses from 27% to a 4% legal maximum. Costs are also reduced by emphasizing disease prevention in place of multi-tiered, crisis medicine. Finally, when a health commissioner with $105 billion to spend negotiates rates and fees with various sectors of the health industry, this practice enables "limiting health care costs" themselves.

The Act declares several rights:

"Californians have a right not to be financially ruined when they or their loved ones become sick or ill.

"California employers have a right not to be driven into insolvency by the spiraling cost of employee medical benefits.

"Californians have a right to high-quality health care.

"Californians should be guaranteed the freedom to choose their own doctor or other health care provider.

"Californians should not be at risk of losing their health benefits if they change or lose their jobs." (25001a-e)[116]

Benefits

It would be bureaucratic to define a list of benefits for all time. Instead, the basic criterion is that a patient gets "all medical care determined to be medically appropriate by the patient's health care provider." (25015) The term "medically appropriate" is common in health care today, and it is broader than what is medically necessary, which is only the minimum required to keep someone alive. The Act does away with interference by insurance companies and managed care reviewers in the doctor-patient relationship; it avoids micro-management by state administrators, too. As we will see, there are global mechanisms for auditing and curbing wasteful medicine, but the Act leaves judgment at the moment of need to the doctor or other health professional.

A provider is not only an M.D. The Act defines a professional provider to be anyone "licensed to provide health care services pursuant to Division 2 of the Business and Professions Code, subject to standards and criteria." (25004z) Licensed chiropractors, acupuncturists, midwives, and mental health professionals may all join the system.

Pharmaceutical drugs are included in the Act's benefits. There will be a "formulary composed of the best-priced prescription drugs of proven efficacy." (25020a) The health commissioner is authorized to use "his or her bidding power to negotiate directly from the manufacturer the lowest possible prices for drugs." (25216a2) The Act does charge "a copayment of not more than five dollars ($5) per prescription" filled in out-patient settings, which is waived for people who do not have the money. (25020d)

The Act supplies **long term care**. It says the health commissioner "shall encourage and reimburse non-institutional long-term services where appropriate." (25025e) The coverage is for attendant care and medical services, but it "shall not cover that portion of long term care expenses incurred for room and board, unless an individual has no resources for payment.... Additional amenities for room and board may be purchased at individual expense." (25025f) It is estimated that in a convalescent home, the uncovered room and board is about 20% of the total bill (55% goes for the medical care and attendance, and 25% for administration).

Long term care is one area where the Act anticipates that people from other states might flock to California and put a financial burden on the plan. The Act basically requires that a person belong to the system for two years before getting benefits for long term care. (25006b) This provision also means that the Act will not begin providing long term care until it has been operating for two years.

Mental health benefits "that are medically appropriate, including, but not limited to, treatment for substance abuse," are provided.

(25030) The Act cautiously phases in coverage. During the first year of the Act, a copayment is charged after 26 out-patient mental health sessions; if the system is not ready to absorb the full cost, the copayment may be renewed one year. (25305b2,c).

Dental benefits are covered only "to the extent funding permits," giving top priority to emergency services, followed by the equivalent of Medicaid coverage, non-cosmetic dentistry for children, and last, care for adults. (25035) The first benefits begin "commencing January 1 of the third year following passage of this Act." (25305d) In effect, the Act wants to get the single payer medical care system up and running smoothly. It anticipates learning how to work more efficiently over the first few years, and then it will have the resources to bring dental care into the system.

Similarly, eyeglasses, hearing aids, and other medical appliances are covered. (25015e) The health commissioner will issue criteria to keep these items a truly medical benefit; Dame Edna cannot expect the fund to pay for her diamond-studded eyeglass frames.

Who Gets a Card?
"All Californians who meet residency requirements defined by the Legislature and certified by the commissioner are eligible for covered benefits." (25006a) Health care is guaranteed for every Californian. We are so used to thinking of health insurance as a privilege that comes with a job or some other economic arrangement that we must train ourselves to grasp health care as a right. A retired person no longer needs to pay Medicare's Part B premiums, its deductibles and copayments. The spouse of a homemaker does not need to ask whether his coverage includes her. There is no such thing as a pre-existing condition that would deny anyone a card.

Children are listed on the card of the adult with legal custody, but a child "who is legally capable of giving consent to health care may apply to the Regional Administrator for a separate card." (25007b2)

A card is not always required. The Act grants presumptive eligibility in certain circumstances. "If a patient arrives at a health facility or clinic who is unconscious, comatose or otherwise unable because of his or her physical or mental condition to document eligibility or to act in his or her own behalf, or if the patient is a minor, the patient shall be presumed to be eligible." (25008)

The Act preserves and expands the state's public health activities, as will be described later. Inoculation campaigns are population-based, which means that they are not recorded through people's health security cards. In other words, if there is an epidemic, everyone is urged to get in line for a shot.

Whether or not someone has a card, "Emergency care and health care services necessary to safeguard the health of the population shall be readily available through the health security system to all individuals." (25059) Local health departments must maintain, with money from the single payer fund, their clinics for underserved groups. (25257b) The Act increases the resources spent on public facilities available to everyone.

Some controversy swirled around the fact that the initiative lets the legislature define who is a state resident for the purpose of getting a health security card. In today's political climate, the Act in effect denies a card to anyone who cannot prove she is here legally. Although the Act devotes additional resources to the safety net that she will continue to use, there will be people with a card and people without one.

On one hand, backers of Proposition 186 did not want to lose voters who would refuse to consider anything pro-immigrant. Complicating the political situation was the presence on the same ballot of an anti-immigrant measure, Proposition 187. As a matter of both conscience and practical politics, almost every active supporter of Proposition 186 opposed Proposition 187. Organizations like Vote Health of Alameda County, a reform group that was one of the backbones of the coalition for Proposition 186, formally endorsed a vote against 187. However, when writing the argument to be included in the voter's guide mailed by the State, CHS's steering committee decided to say that benefits are for "a legal California resident."

Although Proposition 186 helps almost all Latinos, whether "illegal" or not, we do not know yet how many of their votes were lost. In the end, only one well-known group made much noise about residency, the state chapter of the National Organization of Women. First it gave then it withdrew its endorsement of Proposition 186 over the question of health services for immigrants who cannot show they are here legally. However, the whole flap stank of a hidden motive. NOW stuck with its endorsement of Senator Dianne Feinstein. For over a year she had whipped up sentiment against immigrants and made grandstand visits to the California-Mexico border with Attorney General Janet Reno and the border patrol. Just three weeks before the election, a few days after 100,000 Latinos and Asians filled the streets of Los Angeles in anger against Proposition 187, and after William Bennett and Jack Kemp (conservatives who became prominent in the Reagan era) opposed the measure, Feinstein announced against it, too—but only on the grounds that it does not exclude immigrants effectively.

The writers of the Act decided they had to make progress in two steps: first, pass the California Health Security Act. Considering the political temper of 1994, there is no way that a legally sound initiative on health care could pass and prevent the legislature from excluding so-called illegal immigrants. Step two would come later, after the principle of health care as a right had a base of support and a track record of controlling expense. Then a people's movement uniting single payer advocates and defenders of immigrant rights could go back and press the legislature to include everyone who lives on California soil. Meanwhile, many activists worked both for Proposition 186 and against 187.

From Crisis Medicine to Prevention

Preventive medicine covers a variety of activities by which we can stop health problems from occurring and deal with them at earlier rather than later, acute stages.

Unlike the old era of individual physicians (supplemented by underfunded public health services) and the invading corporate regime of managed care, the single payer plan allows a change from crisis medicine to prevention. Everyone is part of one plan and will remain so. Therefore, long term prevention should be expanded enormously, if only for the fiscal incentive that the big payoff of such investments will reduce costs for the health security fund.

The Act has a number of provisions to encourage and require

preventive measures. They range from classic public health for the population as a whole to a long term perspective for the individual patient and her primary care professional.

In its list of basic findings, the Act declares, "Because the best way to control health care costs in the long run is to prevent disease, funding for public health measures, and for research directed at the causes and prevention of disease, should be directly related to the overall cost of illness to society." (25001l) The Act carries out this principle by establishing within the total fund a "Public Health and Prevention Account at a level not less than five percent (5%) of total annual health security system revenues." (25251f2) This amount is at least 30% higher than current state and local public health expenditures, counting the latter as generously as possible.

The public health account pays for campaigns designed to prevent diseases which are "population-based." This term occurs throughout the Act, and it means that public health programs are for all, whether they have a health security card or not. The Act specifically calls for the public health account to "give priority to meeting the population-based health care needs of population groups with the greatest unmet needs, to provide public health outreach to underserved populations." (25251b)

The Act leaves the administration of public health to the state's Department of Health Services; programs may be carried out by grants to local and non-profit agencies, as well as to school-based nurses. (25251d,e)

Besides funding the tasks of public health workers, the Act calls for "specific financial incentives for professional providers to perform community outreach and preventive services." (25210a) In other words, doctors should think about preventive medicine, and the Act connects their income to this job.

An advisory board guides the elected commissioner, and the Act says the board shall consist "of health care and public health professionals and other experts, including the Director of Health Services." (25068a)

The Act specifies that the medical benefits granted to individual holders of a health security card "include outreach, education, and screening services, including, but not limited to: (a) Children's preventive care, well-child care, immunizations, screening, outreach and education. (b) Adult preventive care including mammograms, Pap smears and other screening, outreach, and educational services." (25016)

Today, only one-quarter of newly trained physicians go into primary care. The Act counters, "The people find that quality and efficiency in the delivery of health care services can best be achieved when the ratio of primary care to specialist physicians is one-to-one. Accordingly, the commissioner shall develop and implement appropriate policies which are intended to achieve this ratio." (25260)

Everyone, the Act advises, should have "a designated primary care provider," which may be one person or a group. (25190b) When each cardholder selects one professional, it is better than hopping around with specific complaints from one clinic to another. Although a patient may look around for a doctor whose thinking is in line with her own, she should choose one. The Act defines primary care to mean "comprehensive, longitudinal, individual clinical prevention and treatment services." (25004x) These Latinate syllables declare that it is best when a person goes to one place that knows her history and works with her so that she stays healthy, and together they spot unusual things that may be problems before they become serious.

Paying for the Benefits

When we buy insurance from a corporation, we are customers. If we pool the same amount of money in a public fund, we are taxpayers. "Customer" has a pleasant ring, while the word for our other role has a negative connotation. Conservative politicians complain that a measure would raise taxes, but hardly anyone comments publicly when Prudential or Aetna raises its premiums. The single payer plan can be described as the greatest premium reduction in history. As we examine its finances, we might remember whether some witty guy spoke about taxpayers or customers when he said, "There's one born every minute."

The Act collects the same amount of money that goes today for the health care of the types it will provide, not by premiums and spending out of pocket but through fair taxes. This amount is about $105 billion in 1996, the first year of the Act had it passed on Nov. 8, 1994.

Source of Funds for California Plan ($ billions)

Medicare, other govt. spending	60
Employer payroll tax	34
Individual income tax	10
Tobacco tax	1

Over half the money for the health security fund is already being collected and would fold into the fund. These revenues include Medicare and Medi-Cal (the state's version of Medicaid), money now used for other federal health spending in California, state and local public health funds, and the medical part of the workers' compensation program.

Employers would no longer buy health insurance for their workers. Instead, they would pay a payroll tax at a rate determined by how many full-time equivalent employees they have. (33001)

Payroll Tax by Number of Employees (percent)

Fewer than 10	4.4
From 10 to less than 25	6.0
From 25 to less than 50	7.0
With 50 or more	8.9

The payroll tax reduces expenses for most firms. Small businesses today must figure on 14% of payroll for insurance premiums; large companies spend about 10% plus the cost of administering health benefits. In addition, the levy on all businesses eliminates the cost disadvantage that some companies suffer by buying a policy for their employees while other firms provide nothing.

The payroll tax would raise about $34 billion. It is roughly equal to what employers spend today.

Individuals would not have to buy health insurance nor split a premium with their employer. They would pay a state income tax of 2.5% of taxable income, with a minimum $50 a year per household. (33004) People with very high incomes would pay an additional 2.5%

surtax on the excess over $250,000 per year (for an individual; $500,000 for a married couple). These taxes would supply about $10 billion of the $105 billion total. Three-quarters of taxpayers would pay less for health insurance through the single payer fund than they spend now on premiums and their own outlays for deductibles, copayments, prescription drugs, etc. No one's health policy today matches the comprehensive benefits of the Act.

The individual tax rate created some discussion among people about progressive taxation. Fifty years ago, the term meant levying a higher percentage rate on persons with higher incomes. One justification for a progressive tax was that rich people neither work for their income nor spend all of it; they use a lot of their money to make more money, and they should contribute some of these gains back to society.

In 1994 the argument merely said that someone with a higher income should pay more dollars, although an equal percentage, for the same health benefits as a person with less income. Defenders of the Act tied their argument specifically to health care as a right. A person with average income should not be charged 20% of her wages for health coverage while a rich person spends only 6% of his income. For example, if a family must buy its own health insurance at a cost of $6,000 a year for premiums, this is 20% of the income of a family earning $30,000 (versus a single payer tax of $750) but only 6% for a family earning $100,000 (versus their single payer tax of $2,500).

Apart from the general 2.5% rate, the surtax on high incomes irritated people in opposite ways. It applies only to the excess over $250,000 or $500,000. Some persons felt that it was a tiny vestige of the principle of progressive taxation and should have been stronger. Other people, wanting to attract money from Hollywood liberals, wished that the Act had no graduated tax rates at all.

Finally, the tobacco tax would go up one dollar per pack of cigarettes, raising a token $1 billion. (30123.5)

Cost Control

"It is the intent of the people that expenditures under this Act not exceed in any year expenditures for the prior year adjusted for changes in the state's gross domestic product and population." (25150)

The Act is generously funded. The predictable revenues, plus the savings obtained from eliminating commercial insurance companies and preventing disease, leave a comfortable margin over the known cost of benefits written into the Act. The revenues would average $2,900 per covered person, versus Canada's $,1900; the Kaiser plan delivers its product today with $1,600 per person.

The plan enforces cost control through two methods: global budgeting and specific administrative measures that are available if needed.

Global budgeting is a key element of the single payer plan. "The commissioner, in consultation with the regional administrator, shall prepare a regional budget for each system region. That budget shall include allocations for each of the following: (1) Fee-for-service providers. (2) Capitated providers. (3) Health facilities and associated clinics that are not part of a capitated provider network." (25158)

As mentioned first in the clause, doctors and other health providers may join the system on a fee for service basis. In so doing they agree to uniform fee schedules, which they negotiate annually with the commissioner through their professional groups. The second form of reimbursement, "capitated providers," is the prepaid health plans. A plan, Kaiser for example, agrees to treat each member for a negotiated flat amount per enrollee. The third category includes hospitals, which bargain annually for a facility budget in light of their size and equipment and the expected occupancy rate for their beds. For them, global budgeting saves the administrative overhead of billing every aspirin to a policy claim against one or another of 1,200 insurance companies.

The health commissioner and the various players in the health industry know that for the coming year Californians will have so many babies, need so many bones set, develop so many cases of hepatitis, etc. The rates and fees, multiplied by the statistically predictable frequency of tasks, cannot exceed the money in the fund. As over two decades of Canadian experience show, global negotiations are completed every year. Of course, some doctors and health industry executives may be unhappy about losing opportunities to boost charges; they might decide to leave medicine and go into investment banking. Farewell!

Global budgeting is the opposite of the main technique employed by commercial insurance companies following the model of corporatized medicine ("managed care"). They use their control of the claims process to intrude non-professionals into the doctor-patient relationship. The single payer system has no case reviewers asking a physician why Jane Doe is still in the hospital four days after her operation.

Could a physician "churn the system"? Yes, he could get away with a few cases, and the single payer plan allows that to happen for the greater good of letting professionals exercise their judgment. However, the following hypothetical scenario illustrates how the health commissioner can deal with financial abuse. Suppose she notices that births by Caesarian operation have a statistical profile that divides in two: 30% of the obstetricians have a low rate of Caesarians, while 70% perform them twice as often. (We have made up exaggerated percentages.) Furthermore, outcomes show little difference in the babies' health. When the commissioner discusses next year's fees for delivering a baby, she lays out this information and suggests that the obstetricians need to review their guidelines for Caesarians. She presumably has backing from the 30% of doctors who pay more attention to the Hippocratic oath than to their stock portfolio. Of course, for the really bad apples, "An individual provider whose billing volume or distribution suggests the possibility of impropriety may be subject to investigation by the commissioner…and may be subject to exclusion or other penalties" such as fines of not more than $5,000 per violation. (25196b, 25286)

As observed in an earlier chapter, Canadian doctors earn comfortable incomes, although not at the same high multiple of an average worker's earning as a physician in the United States. The scenario above indicates that health professionals will be rewarded enough to attract them to the field, but an active health commissioner can promote an ethical climate of honesty and service.

Although global budgeting is the main tool of cost control, the Act has additional remedies for curbing specific costs.

The advisory board may "identify medical services for which there is no credible evidence of significant benefit." (25070e)

> "Restrictions on, and copayments for, elective services, as
> necessary to balance the system budget, shall be applied by the

commissioner in order of increasing efficacy, as determined by the advisory board, in order that those elective services that are clearly beneficial for treatment of a patient's condition be the last services to be restricted or to have a copayment applied." (25240c) The commissioner may exclude coverage of a specific diagnosis if her advisory board finds "that the diagnosis or the available treatments are often inappropriate." (25240d1)

"The commissioner shall not carry out any cost control measure that limits access to care that is needed on an emergent or urgent basis, or that is medically appropriate for treatment of a patient's medical condition." (25225)

We must remember that the essence of the single payer plan is health care without insurance companies, hence savings in administration, marketing, and profiteering. The removal of the insurance companies has consequences throughout the health industry. For example, the largest section in most hospitals is the billing department. California hospitals spend over 20% of their budgets on administration. A hospital has a much reduced burden of paperwork dealing with one single payer fund rather than 1,200 insurance companies. More important, the hospital's battle for claims payment fought with the micromanagers of the insurance companies ends. Administration should take about what it takes a Canadian hospital, 9%.[117]

It might seem that giving health security to six million Californians who have no insurance today goes on the books as an expansion of cost, pure and simple. This is not correct. When everyone has a health security card, much treatment that occurs now in emergency rooms will happen in the office of a primary care doctor, and earlier in the course of illness rather than at a moment of crisis. Savings result from relocating treatment out of the most expensive place for it, the emergency room, as well as from earlier, simpler, less lengthy care performed by a family doctor instead of by a specialist.

"We Want Our Plan Run This Way"

One way that we can understand how the people govern their single payer plan and have public servants administer it is by comparing the model set up in the Act with the way bosses run insurance corporations.

Although the chief executive officer (CEO) of a corporation supposedly answers to a board of directors, it is his show as long as the company generates good profits on the capital invested by the owners. He enjoys huge pay, bonuses and stock options, and the comforts of office for an indefinite number of years, usually until retirement. Only if a serious crisis of profits requires major changes and the CEO is too lazy or unwilling to make them, might the board of directors or a group of large shareholders oust him.

As for his relation to holders of health insurance policies, the CEO is too high and mighty to deal with any one individual among them, and the idea of a collective of customers making themselves heard is simply unthinkable. Premiums, unlike taxes, are not items of discussion. The rule is, if you don't like our terms, take your few dollars somewhere else.

Doctors working in an HMO or signed up on a network of preferred providers have slightly more say with the insurance organization. They have usually joined the group under the pressure of the market: everyone else is running for referrals into a network, so I had better do the same. This economic compulsion is masked, at least for a few years, by high salaries and bonuses as well as the superficial appearance of respect and consultation. However, physicians slowly lose their professional medical autonomy and fill a slot in a non-medical organization. The insurance company, directed from the top by the goal of increased return on capital, has more to tell the doctor every day about how she will practice and deliver health care.

The non-counterpart to the CEO in the California Health Security Act is a health commissioner. "The commissioner shall stand for election at the same time and in the same manner as the Governor." (25060b) However, "The first commissioner shall be appointed by the Governor not less than 75 nor more than 100 days following passage of this act, and shall be confirmed by the Legislature within 30 days of nomination." (25060c)

Neither the commissioner, her family, nor any of the other major officials to be described shortly, may have "a financial interest in the outcome of deliberations in which that member would participate as a result of their appointment, during the time of appointment and for a period of three years after completion of the appointment." (25060j)

The commissioner appoints an advisory board of health care and public health professionals (25065c1), a deputy commissioner (25060i), regional administrators for system regions which bring the working of the single payer plan closer to people, and regional consumer advocates for each region (25065c2,3). The consumer advocates investigate complaints, referring cases as needed to a licensing board or law enforcement agencies. (25075c) The advocates also hold annual public hearings and publish an annual report conveying complaints and suggestions from the public and reviewing the health facilities in the region and their performance. (25075d)

How much will the administrative apparatus cost? When we compare overhead expenses from existing experience, the advantage of a single payer plan over commercial insurance corporations is clear. Canada's provincial and federal governments together spend less than 2% on administrative overhead. Medicare in the U.S. spends 2%. Private insurers spend 14% on administration, but a total of 27% adding in marketing and sales commissions.[118]"Commencing with the second budget year, the administrative costs of the health security system incurred by the commissioner shall be 4 percent or less of the total funds appropriated for the health security system. If administrative costs exceed this target, the commissioner shall report to the Legislature the reasons for excess administrative costs." (25175)

The conceptual equation for health reform is: single payer = public insurance + private health care. Once she has a health security card, a California resident interacts with doctors, clinics, and health plans, not with a state agency like the department of motor vehicles. Perhaps she will receive a mailing about an anti-flu inoculation campaign or see a billboard purchased by the single payer system urging pregnant women to get prenatal care. Contrary to scare cries of government bureaucracy, she does not wait in line to see a state clerk. She simply goes to the physician, clinic, or Kaiser or other health plan of her choice.

While individual consumers do not deal with a state office, they have the opportunity to join a public debate over policy that no insurance CEO tolerates. This happens because the plan sets up an independent consumer council. Consumer rights advocates working in Ralph Nader's group wrote this portion of the Act.

"The membership of the consumer council shall consist of all individual health care consumers 16 years of age or older residing in the state who have contributed to the consumer council the appropriate annual membership fee. The Board of Directors of the Health Care Consumer Council shall establish an annual membership fee of not less than ten dollars ($10), to be adjusted every three years for inflation, and provide for reduced fee membership for low income individuals." (25080b)

Suppose one million Californians take the voluntary decision to join the consumer council, giving it an independent budget of $10 million. It speaks out on health insurance policy, educates cardholders about their rights, and conducts research and surveys. (25080a) The Act requires, "The commissioner shall make available to the consumer council all available information regarding administration and any other aspects of the health security system." (25090g) What managed care plan would open its books to a patients' council?

The Act requires annual public hearings in each region to take testimony on budget matters, health policies, and the performance of hospitals and clinics. The consumer council is written into the Act as a joint sponsor with the commissioner of these hearings. (25090)

A board of directors governs the consumer council, 20 of 25 members being elected from around the state. (25080e) The council cannot endorse political parties or candidates for elective office. (25080n)

We already described how doctors and other health care providers relate to the system through bargaining with the commissioner. These talks arrive at uniform rates and fees every year. While the commissioner has great power on behalf of all Californians, the provider groups have more opportunity for give and take than they do with managed care plans and insurance companies. One reason is that groups of physicians, specialists of various kinds, chiropractors, hospital associations, and other providers can bargain as groups, speaking with one voice for their profession or sector of the health industry. The

Act declares the intent of the people that the bargaining groups be exempt from antitrust laws. (25520)

The elected health commissioner, unlike the CEO of an insurance company, is not guided by the profit motive. Instead, her official goal is to provide the best universal health care within the constraint of resources that are fixed as a portion of the whole economy. She has the powers necessary to carry out the job, and she is one responsible person, not a legislature and governor whose members and parties say, "I tried to get my bill passed, but gridlock prevented it."

Favoring public oversight is the fact that health care is the subject of the agency. People take more interest in the terms of their health insurance and how they are treated than they do in, for example, the technical details of setting electricity rates by the public utilities commission.

As noted, the commissioner cannot have a financial interest in the health system, and her pay does not separate her from the ordinary citizen like those of corporate CEOs. She might well have an eye set on higher office. In any event, she must submit to election in an environment of public hearings and informed review by a consumer group.

Transition and Other Details

The Act starts providing benefits on "January 1 of the second year following passage of this act." (25305a) If the Act had passed on Nov. 8, 1994, the single payer fund would have opened for business on Jan. 1, 1996. The Act addresses several questions about the transition to health care without insurance companies and about changing the terms of the Act itself as the march of events will require.

Retraining. The finances of the California Health Security Act are "economy neutral." It shifts money from insurance company waste to a full package of health care for more Californians, but the spending and the number of jobs should be about the same. However, the work will be different. Insurance companies are notorious for unrewarding clerical jobs. For the transition, it is a good thing that turnover is high.

The Act sets up "for a period of at least three years after benefits are first provided, a Health Worker Training Account." Its funding is "equal to one percent (1%) of the system budget, unless the commissioner determines that a different amount is needed for prudent operation of the health security system." Job retraining and apprenticeships help "health workers displaced by transition to the health security system to be retrained and placed in jobs that meet the new needs of the system." The commissioner may propose to extend the retraining account in her budgets after three years. (25255)

Long term care in particular, which the Act encourages to be in the patient's home when possible, should create a large demand for qualified attendants.

Retired employees with benefits. Some retired workers have health insurance supplied by their former employer. The retirees wondered how they would fare under Proposition 186. One big benefit of the Act is that the retiree would not have to take out an expensive policy ($1,500 or more per person) for long term care—or risk bankruptcy and poverty by not having such a policy and perhaps needing long term care at some later date. They would not have to pay $500 a year for Medicare Part B, which is today's premium charge for doctor services (Part A covering hospital services has no premium). They would not need a supplemental policy to cover Medicare's growing number of deductibles and payout limits.

Policies for retirees of private employers typically have deductibles, copayments, and uncovered costs like prescription drugs. The retiree's health security card provides full health care without these charges.

Adding it all up, the 2.5% on taxable income is a good deal for any retiree with less than $100,000 income.

In the system or outside it. Both insurance companies and physicians are free to continue doing business outside the single payer plan, although few would find it worthwhile.

The Act avoids much potential harassment in court by not regulating health insurance companies. They may continue to offer policies. The only rule is that the company must tell prospective customers "in writing of the benefits for which they may be eligible under the health security system." The commissioner may set the wording and type size of a notice that must be displayed in the ad and policy. (25415) Any Californian who wants to buy a policy duplicating benefits that are hers by right may do so.

Physicians and other providers who join the single payer plan (a decision that is completely their own (25420)) shall "not charge the patient any additional amount" (except for system-set copayments). (25180a3) This rule prevents the revival of multi-tier medicine within the single payer fund. A doctor cannot accept money from the fund and add a surcharge to patients who might be willing to pay. The Act gives everyone in the society from top to bottom an interest in maintaining a single standard of care for herself and everyone else.

As for services not covered under the Act, like most cosmetic procedures, a physician may perform the service for any customer who wants to pay. (25421b)

The Act and the legislature. The initiative submitted to the voters on Nov. 8, 1994, would have changed California statutory law. It also would have added a few lines to the state constitution in order to separate the health security fund from the general fund and the rest of California state finances. (Sections 3, 4) Some people are not happy with detailed initiatives in place of deliberations through the legislature. Normally, the League of Women Voters takes this view. However, the California LWV not only endorsed Proposition 186 but also made it the group's number one legislative priority for the year.

The Act's provisions are difficult, easy, or impossible for the legislature to change. The general rule demands a two-thirds vote of the membership of the legislature; any change in the tax rates falls under this requirement. (Section 9) It takes only a majority vote to pass legislation that implements the Act, for example, folding workers' compensation into the single payer fund. Finally, the legislature cannot change the intent of the Act even by a unanimous vote. The detailed findings and purposes stated at the beginning of the Act are therefore protected from legislative tampering. Citizens may sue to overturn a legislative amendment, although they have the burden of proving that the amendment is inconsistent with the purposes and findings. (25400)

One item of transition that the Act failed to address is how to dispose of the insurance companies' contingency funds. Insurers maintain reserves to pay future health claims by policyholders. When the single payer fund takes over the obligation for care, it has a right to this money, too. Alternatively, the Act might liquidate the reserves by specifying a refund to policyholders. People got a hint of the amounts at stake when Blue Cross in California set up a for-profit company, Wellpoint, and supplied it with funds that grew tax-free for decades at the expense of the public. Without independent audit, Blue Cross admitted that such reserves are at least $2.5 billion.

6

Class Interests For and Against Reform

What do social groups gain and lose under different proposals for health care reform? The political economy largely works out to a contrast between the single payer plan on one hand and all the rest, which leave health care under the rule of insurance corporations. These include the schemes of Clinton and the market-based reformers. Variations of the latter are important to employers and providers, and they produce splits and gridlock in Washington.

Insurance Companies

Twenty-five years ago the Canadians adopted a single payer plan before corporate profit interests had a big, lucrative health care business. Today U.S. insurance companies and other powers of corporatized medicine are dug in, spending tens of millions of dollars in order to frustrate reform that would eliminate multi-billion dollar lines of business.

While the largest insurance corporations have the resources to dominate the managed care industry, the majority of the 1,200 health insurance companies do not. This difference gives rise to a political split. As we saw, the big five favored legislation that promotes their managed care plans. To them, universal coverage means requiring by law that every American pay them premiums. It means forcing all but the wealthiest persons to enroll in a plan chosen from a short list.

The Health Insurance Association of America, speaking for the rest of the insurance companies, prefers as little change as possible from the current situation. This clash between insurers was behind much of the backdoor wrangling in Congress. The insurance companies bought politicians, which is delicately called lobbying. Then Prop. 186 came up in California. The HIAA sent $1.5 million to oppose it, while the big five's Alliance for Managed Competition contented itself with less than $900,000.[119]

Insurance companies buy television time, and they use their muscle to exclude other points of view. Starting in May 1993, the group Neighbor to Neighbor attempted to run 30-second television commercials in favor of the single payer plan. Station executives refused to put the $2,000 spot on the air, explaining that it would risk loss of much more revenue from insurance companies.[120]

The insurance companies suppressed media explanation of single payer at the start of the national discussion. Although the single payer alternative has wide sympathy among the public and had nearly 100 sponsors in Congress, a computer search found that ABC's *World News Tonight* mentioned it once during the entire year of 1993.[121]

After the boundaries of so-called realistic reform were set, the corporate media tolerated occasional mentions of the single payer plan, especially since many of its sponsors merely used it as a bargaining chip to modify the Clinton and other proposals. In July 1994, the NBC network gave ten minutes of a two-hour program on health reform to the single payer advocates. Viewers were also treated to the spectacle of Senator Robert Dole saying that individual states should be free to adopt single payer, even though he thought the concept was a bad one. A few weeks later, of course, Dole gave his tacit support to amendments that would make single payer plans in the states more difficult to set up and administer.

The businessmen of health bought off some of their individual opponents, too. Single payer advocate David Himmelstein, M.D., reports, "The AFL's health policy director [Karen M. Ignagni] slid easily into leadership of the HMOs' trade association; Citizen Action's chief moved to a job selling the Clinton plan for the Democratic National Committee."[122]

All insurance companies are dead set against the single payer plan, because it would make health care a right for everyone and remove almost all commercial policies from the scene as useless.

The Rest of Big Capital
Big capital helped put health care on the country's political agenda.

Certain corporations were especially concerned about their cost. Companies were more likely to be upset if they faced international competition, since other countries get better health care for less money and spread the cost through their societies. Companies obligated to a large base of retirees and staffed by older workforces, like the automobile manufacturers, have costs higher than companies who do not promise retiree benefits and have younger employees, such as anti-union Apple Computer and big retailers.

Five years ago, sections of big capital were ready to control costs by turning to the federal government. "I never thought I would be in favor of a government health policy, but there are things that government must do. We have to spread the burden," said Robert E. Mercer, just retired as chairman of Goodyear Tire and Rubber. Basically, he wanted Medicare expanded to take over expenses that big companies paid through family benefits and as a target of cost-shifting within the health industry. A spokesman for a group of 180 corporations sounded reluctantly radical: "There is grudging recognition...that health care has moved to being a right."[123] These attitudes would change when managed care plans offered cost control.

Fast food chains like PepsiCo and General Mills, and other business that use part time workers at low wages and with high turnover, do not want to provide any benefits to employees. Even if the companies all had to pay a payroll tax so that no one corporation had a cost edge over the others, the fast food industry competes with supermarkets and does not want to give them a level playing field.

So far the conflict of interests among big corporations has been mild. Their executives have sympathy with each other. Insurers tie corporations together through large investments and interlocking directors. David M. Roderick, a director of Aetna Life & Casualty, is also on the boards of Procter & Gamble, Texas Instruments, and USX Corp. Edward H. Budd, chairman and CEO of The Travelers Corp., chats with his colleagues on the boards of directors at Delta Air Lines and GTE Corp. Cigna Corp. director Robert P. Bauman is also on the boards at Capital Cities/ABC Inc. and Union Pacific, and he is the CEO at Smithkline Beecham.[124]

The Business Roundtable came out against Clinton's plan and in favor of more raw market power for insurers. This group of the top

200 corporations was content to let an insurance company executive lead the study committee that produced their legislative stand.

Big capital sees that commercial managed care plans may well slow down cost increases by cutting service to patients and the wages of health workers, and that is satisfactory to corporate chiefs. For most of them, the ideal solution to the health crisis has three features. First, it reduces medical inflation, because health care simply eats up too much of the economy, especially in comparison with other countries. Second, it relieves big employers of the burden they feel as a result of cost-shifting. They see their insurance premiums subsidizing the uninsured, because hospitals and the medical industry generally raise charges to the insured in order to make up for the uninsured.

Third, an ideal solution for big capital keeps multi-tier medicine and job-connected health benefits. Employers like to have benefits on the table along with wages. If a single payer system takes health plans out of bargaining, the employees, whether negotiating collectively or individually, are free to concentrate on their pay and working conditions. The employer much prefers a situation where workers must decide between wage demands and health benefits.

Furthermore, multi-tier medicine goes along with a basic capitalist principle for the labor market—inequality. Put a different price on the labor of different people, and buy only the degree of skill or commitment that the employer needs. If the employer can offer health benefits that look good by comparison with the rest of the marketplace, he can attract the skilled people and demand the commitment he needs for certain positions. For other jobs, the employer simply keeps the total wage as low as possible. It helps if he does not pay for health benefits, or pays for minimal benefits, but certainly he does not want to pay a payroll tax on every job. He does not like to bargain with an employee who reminds him of her individual income tax that finances public health insurance for everyone.

Big capital is class conscious. The chiefs of huge corporations, Wall Street investment banks, and their top lawyers and political agents do not make decisions by numbers. Certainly, they want so-called hard data, but unlike the ordinary engineer who calculates the efficiency and cost of technical alternatives, the men of big capital know that struggle between classes helps make the numbers. It is impossible for reformers to sell a single payer plan to big capital by submitting data proving its cost effectiveness. These men know that an institutional change could limit their power and stimulate labor activism and popular demands for more reform.

Although inequality on the labor market is a general capitalist principle, the distinction between big and small capital sometimes obscures it. Big capital is content to let small business fight a battle against a social reform. Yet many small firms exist as suppliers and subcontractors to big corporations. For example, computer firms with an image like Apple Computer contract assembly work to sweatshops like Solectron and little garage operations. Such smaller businesses exist because they engage in management by high pressure, they have no "corporate culture" to maintain, and they can function with high turnover that is cumbersome for large companies. The owners of these businesses sense, if they do not fully realize, that they have an economic niche only because they take advantage of the principle of labor inequality in a specific way.

As goes economic relations, so go politics. When reforms attack the interest of capital in general, big capital often stays behind the scenes while small business comes out as the unpopular but "realistic" voice of "the market," which cannot tolerate minimum standards of human existence. In Dec. 1990 San Francisco adopted a mild law enforcing safety standards for employees who use video display terminals. Companies had four years to adjust lighting so that workers do not develop eye trouble and to arrange furniture and keyboards so that people's wrists do not become bundles of crippled, painful nerves and muscle. But two small office firms (Data Processing & Accounting Services and Zack Electronics) filed suit against the law. It turned out that the companies, both doing business with IBM, could afford to sue because the corporation gave them money for the litigation. The Service Employees International Union Local 790 was particularly upset when it discovered IBM's financial backing, because the union had agreed to a watered-down ordinance in return for a pledge that big business would not challenge it.[125]

During the 1994 battle over health reform in Washington, the insurance companies and other parts of corporatized medicine had the most immediate economic interests and fought for them with tens of millions of dollars in lobbying, TV campaigns, and legalized bribery. Large corporations spoke up to the degree that their particular situations demanded reform. Some wanted employer mandates, others did not. But no one in big capital seriously pushed Rep. McDermott's single payer bill.

When Californians took up a single payer initiative, the insurance companies bankrolled the opposition, as we will see, and let small business groups like the Chamber of Commerce be the front men. The rest of big capital opposed single payer reform mostly by inertia. They did not endorse Proposition 186. Some of them attacked it in newsletters to employees.

A vocal exception, Hewlett-Packard, spoke out publicly against the measure, saying that it would cost the company $60 million a year. This corporation, praised for wonderful management and corporate culture, spends less than 6% of payroll on health benefits.[126] Many of the company's California employees are young, highly paid professionals, while H-P does its manufacturing out of state and overseas. An H-P engineer was left widowed and $220,000 in debt after his wife, also an H-P engineer, spent months in the hospital fighting lupus disease unsuccessfully. She exhausted a $500,000 lifetime limit on her supposedly gold-plated benefits.

Big capital will accept health reform under certain conditions. Canada is a capitalist country. So is the United Kingdom, which adopted nationalized health care. Capital has learned to live with social democratic reforms across most of western Europe, too (never in total peace, always looking for ways to undermine accomplishments and reverse trends). People will find out exactly what big capital in the U.S. will do when they push forward their struggle for health care as a right.

Small Business

The divisions within small business can be sharp. Before various economic interests dug into unyielding political positions, a 1989 survey of the bosses of 565 small companies responded on national health insurance 38% in favor, 39% against, and 23% undecided.[127]

For reasons explained above, some small business owners oppose all reforms, whether it is a mandate that the employer provide the weakest of benefits or the payroll tax of a single payer plan. The National Federation of Independent Businesses speaks for these diehard opponents of all change.

On the other hand, a small employer who wants his staff to be healthy and free of worry can appreciate a solution at the ballot box. It covers him and his competitors all at once, instead of making him take on costs to his disadvantage.

Other small businesses will want a single payer plan because it is the only one that really controls costs. The employer would find it a relief not to deal with relentless annual rate increases. Many owners, comparing the graduated payroll tax in the California Health Security Act to their current and likely premium charges, recognized that the single payer plan is cheaper by one- to two-thirds. In addition, rates for worker's compensation will go down, and the medical portions of auto and liability insurance become unnecessary.

Furthermore, small employers fear that the insurer will cancel the policy if anyone in the company should be so bold as actually to use the benefits. Large employers who deliver a broad base for cost averaging do not have this problem. The single payer plan would put an end to worry over cancellation.

Boutique businesses have a few, highly skilled employees whose dedication is essential for success of the firm; they sell to customers who, although interested in price, need quality work they cannot perform themselves. Such firms tend to be the strongest supporters of solving the health care crisis. On the other hand, a company that begs one or two large corporations for contract assembly jobs and has only price to offer is likely to oppose the single payer plan. Even if the owner and his competitors all have to pay, he is afraid that his customer corporation will take jobs in-house and automate them.

Although they are not profit-making businesses, schools, cities, and other units of local government would obtain the same relief as every employer. The payroll tax of 8.9% is less than the typical bill currently paid to the insurance companies for health premiums. For example, California school districts would have saved $600 million under Proposition 186. They would have money to pay the employees' 2.5% income tax and some left over.

The Working Class

For two centuries workers have struggled for a better life, fighting both at the workplace and in the political arena. The work hours of a day were the subject of great movements, in England for the ten-hour day and later in the nineteenth century in the United States for the eight-hour day. To take another example, the pre-Civil War era named for President Andrew Jackson was as much a time of labor political movements and parties; one of their major issues went beyond the problems of the workshop and raised the demand for public education of their children not as "a grace and bounty or charity" but as "a matter of right."[128] (Reactionaries did not have the communist label then, so they denounced "Workeyism.")

Health care as a right is nothing less than a chapter of this labor tradition which is in play now, not in history books but before our eyes. In past decades workers fought for health benefits attached to the job. The gains of this struggle are real but always incomplete and unstable. The individual worker loses her benefits if she loses her job, which ironically might happen because a disease makes it impossible for her to work. She must figure every potential change of job by comparing not only wages and other satisfactions but also the health benefits, which might be lost totally if she has a pre-existing condition. When health care comes with a job, the move from active work to retirement becomes a source of worry, because retirement benefits are a separate issue again.

During World War II and for two decades after it, U.S. workers increased their health benefits. In many negotiations and strikes they won health insurance partly at the cost of plain wage gains. Lately, workers are in a defensive posture, and the major issue in three strike actions out of four from 1989 to 1992 was health care benefits.[129]The first thing every employer puts on the table is a bigger copayment and a higher deductible, restricted choice of health plans, less coverage for the spouse and children, reduced benefits in retirement, and other takebacks. Whether the workers defeat them or not, they are weaker when talks get around to pay and working conditions. We can hardly estimate how much employees gave up in potential wage gains or in outright concessions in order to maintain health care.

The single payer plan removes health care from the bargaining table and makes it a right that a worker keeps regardless of unemployment, retirement, job switch, and change in marriage situation. The single payer plan guarantees security for the millions of workers whose employers do not provide a health policy. As proposed by the California Health Security Act, the benefits cover health needs like no commercial insurance policy, including long term care.

The average working person would pay less and get more coverage with a single payer plan. Under the California Health Security Act, for example, she pays 2.5% of her taxable income (not gross income). With a taxable income of $35,000, the amount works out to $73 a month. In return, she pays no insurance premium and deductibles. For many people this calculation would decide the issue in favor of single payer right away, as compared to the employee's 20% to 50% share of a basic premium, estimated to be $1,900 for an individual or $4,300 for a family on average, and going up rapidly.

Many established labor leaders have stuck with another solution, proposals like the original Clinton plan that required every employer to provide benefits, supplemented by extending Medicaid or Medicare to the unemployed. The method of employer mandates is neither workable nor acceptable, for three reasons. First, employers purchase policies from commercial insurance companies, and experience shows that it is impossible to guarantee everyone health care at a cost that the economy can bear so long as the insurance companies, with their waste and market games and profiteering, dominate health insurance.

Second, mandates retain multi-tier medicine in the patchwork of employer and government channels for providing health care. Multi-tier medicine inevitably means insufficient care for broad sections of the population.

Third, nothing in the method of employer mandates embodies the right of health care in an institution. The problem that immediately arises with employer mandates is the "portability" of a person's health insurance, and the change in benefit level, as she moves to a different job, is laid off, or retires. It is unclear how a patchwork system will keep track of changes in one's status relating to multiple sellers of health insurance, employment-based coverage, and government help between jobs. A worker would keep her health security card, but every doctor, hospital, and health center would need to check that the card is valid, that an insurance policy from an employer or a government agency is in effect at the moment she arrives for treatment. By contrast, the single payer plan has one fund, and everyone's health security card is valid simply because it confers a universal right.

Besides noting matters of principle, workers with a trade union have a petty influence to throw off, too. Some labor leaders, like the head of the building trades department of the AFL-CIO, wear a second hat, chief of an insurance fund. As bit players in the industry who would lose a position when the single payer plan goes into effect, they have a split in interest from their members.

When an advocate proposes a single payer solution, employees among the shrinking category of those who still have health plans paid entirely by the employer ask, do you want me to pay a new 2.5% income tax? Yes. The benefits are better, including long term care. The single payer plan guarantees security beyond your current employment. You might not be aware of limits and exclusions in the fine print of your policy, and employers continually change the terms of their gift to you.

It is true that employees in comparatively good situations today will need to go through a round of bargaining for the transition to a single payer plan. The employer will save money when he switches from commercial policies to the payroll tax capped at 8.9%. He stops the expense of administering health coverage, too. The employees, in a trade union or individually, must argue like this: you provide good benefits because you want dedicated workers who are not distracted by worry about the potential of medical disasters, so we want a raise to cover our 2.5% income tax. Once this transition is made, workers enjoy stronger bargaining in the future because health care is off the table.

Much of this discussion has been about workers who bargain collectively. It applies to employees and prospective hires who negotiate individually with an employer for pay and benefits, too. These talks depend on the general state of the labor market.

Some categories of the working class have a special interest in the single payer plan because it makes health care a right for everyone. Part time and temporary workers will have benefits in full. Many persons who are formally self-employed really sell their ability to labor and nothing else; their contracts with one firm after another amount to employment situations. They, too, will get health care.

These sections of the working class blend into the smallest of small business. They are working people, and the advantages of a single payer plan are theirs, too.

Other groups created by the ravages of an oppressive economy are those who are more or less permanently unemployed, as well as women struggling to raise a family without a partner. Health care as a right is vital for them. They would have the same health security card as everyone else. Unlike Medicaid, no government office would run them through hoops to verify eligibility for each incident of treatment. Nor would a recipient lose health care when she obtained a job and began to earn a halfway decent income. Furthermore, the single payer plan embraces diverse health care providers, including public clinics and county-run general hospitals. California's Proposition 186 would have given them new funds.

Some state and county governments want to contract out their Medicaid responsibilities to managed care plans run for profit. This scheme would strengthen multi-tier medicine. HMOs specializing in Medicaid patients would operate far differently than plans aimed at upscale clientele. For example, the plan would drag its feet on referral to an appropriate specialist or facility that is not on the plan's core roster. Regardless of the frustrations in the public setup today, people on Medicaid do not want to be herded into such managed care plans, and the single payer alternative is the best of all.

Finally, a political reason for workers to lead the fight for a single payer plan deserves mention: it will unite people and promote a revived movement that changes the political atmosphere of the country.

Senior Citizens

Medicare recipients would gain with a single payer plan. They would get the same comprehensive benefits as everyone else in place of the eroding provisions of Medicare. They would not pay Medicare Part B, nor would they buy a Medigap policy and worry about premium hikes. The California Health Security Act would have given senior citizens (and all of us) prescription drugs and phased in long term care, too. No alternative comes close to such health security.

Still, recipients bring their experience with Medicare to their evaluation of a new public scheme, the single payer plan. On one hand, recipients have come to know their way around Medicare. They certainly do not want it taken away, and they must assure themselves that in a single payer plan the process of getting care really is easier, cheaper, and more secure. Once someone has a health security card, she does not worry about renewing her card nor about verifying that Part B is in force. On the other hand, recipients wonder if typical Medicare frustrations would continue: finding a physician who takes Medicare patients (an overrated problem) and accepts Medicare's fee schedule, and getting government actually to pay the bill. In a single payer plan, all doctors automatically take any health cardholder, and they have already agreed through a professional group on a schedule of reimbursement. The bill goes directly from provider to the single payer fund; the patient is out of this loop entirely.

Even before the congressional elections of 1994, a diverse collection of big capital's opinion servants complained that entitlements cost too much. Now there is even more open talk about so-called Medicare savings. Senior citizens would enjoy much greater security with a fund of the kind in California's plan. It largely escapes the annual budget wrangling of a legislature or Congress. Also, while seniors are a powerful interest group, a single payer fund has a much broader range of people who benefit and will defend it. Reactionaries would find it harder to roll out the vicious tactic of pitting young against old, for example.

Retired people with health plans from their former employer understandably wanted to investigate and resolve concerns about a single payer plan. As discussed in the previous chapter, their coverage would expand, most notably for long term care, and it would be more secure than the changing roster of plans and terms offered by the former employer.

Sectors of Health Care

Apart from insurers, participants in the health industry divide along the same general class lines as the economy in general.

Hospitals lobby for their special interest and generally oppose the single payer plan. Some administrators enjoy the marketplace in which they have prospered. Others are on the prowl like HMO executives and think they can be winning businesses in the new world of managed care. All of them aim to expand their empires, and they want nothing to do with the global budgeting of a single payer plan.

Hospitals and other health care institutions are highly political beings. Early in 1994 some politicians suggested that the marketplace had already begun to curb runaway medical inflation. It peaked at 9.7% in 1991 and by the end of 1993 had fallen to a rate of 4.4%, the lowest in 20 years.[130] However, this pattern has occurred several times. Health care rises to the top of the national agenda, the increase of medical charges slows down, the issue passes, and then price hikes resume. Figures on the growth of health spending, adjusted to remove general inflation, show the history.

In the early 1970s, health care becomes an issue

1972	9%
1973	3
1974	2

Reform proposal dies in Congress

1975	5
1976	8
1978	5

President Carter proposes universal coverage, cost caps

1979	1

Reagan elected[131]

1980	1
1981	5
1983	7

Physicians are torn one way and the other, sometimes with so much tension that they doubt their choice of career.

A few are money-hungry entrepreneurs, seeking their pot of gold in the unsettled marketplace, launching managed care networks and other businesses. A few more become executives for big ventures in corporatized medicine.

Many doctors, particularly certain specialists, get not merely good but very high incomes. Even as the supply of specialists grew during the 1980s, the average income of a physician, excluding residents in training, swelled 21% after inflation from 1983 to 1990. In 1991 their average earnings were $170,000. Doctors may want to keep their income high and rising, but it will not be easy. HMOs dangle juicy rewards to become part of the operation, but physicians sense that five years down the road they may need to fight their new corporate masters. Many HMOs already limit doctors' income. On the other hand, as HMOs take over more of medicine, the practitioner who finds customers on his own and charges a fee for service must contend with strong competition.

Managed care plans run a squeeze on their primary care doctors under which they remain nominally independent businessmen but are worse off in some ways than salaried employees. The plan pays the physician an annual amount for each patient that it sends him from its rolls. At the same time, the company penalizes the doctor for excessive referrals to specialists. The physician delivers considerable treatment in his office facilities. He ramps up capacity as the plan draws him into its network, but he may be stuck with excess capacity if the plan cancels the contract and takes away his client roster. Concerning patients, one doctor bluntly described how managed care companies do business: "In fiscal terms, patients have become salable capital assets of health plans that essentially loan them on consignment to physicians."[132]

As for a single payer fund, some independent doctors do not like the idea of their medical society negotiating a binding, public fee schedule with the state health commissioner. Yet in their single payer plan, Canadian physicians have maintained generous incomes. One attractive feature of the system is that it gets rid of insurance company interference in the practice of medicine. Many hours per week of paperwork and politely hostile telephone conversations about treatment decisions would disappear. Office overhead would be reduced.

About 7,000 doctors joined together in Physicians for a National Health Program and endorsed a single payer plan. The National Medical Association (representing African-American physicians) and the Women's Medical Association favor single payer, too. The American College of Surgeons, which has 53,000 members, told a Congressional hearing that it supports nationalized health insurance in principle.[133] The *Journal of the AMA* regularly accepts articles arguing that a single payer plan helps the practice of medicine.

Health care workers, the broad ranks of nurses, attendants, and service staff in hospitals and health centers, can appreciate anything that restrains the profit motive in medicine. These workers face continual attacks on their trade unions, their wages and benefits, and job security. The single payer movement contends with the profiteers of corporatized medicine, the insurance and managed care companies, for the direction of health care in the twenty-first century.

Nurses in particular have proved to be enthusiastic advocates of a single payer solution. Very few of them have the opportunity dangled in front of some physicians to join the top ranks of executives out for their pot of gold. But nurses have as much professional and human concern for their patients as physicians. Nurses see the substance of their work, rooted in the history of the occupation, under attack.

Hospital managers want to replace registered nurses by unskilled and quickly trained labor. Many jobs for R.N.'s would disappear, while the remainder, taken away from the patient's bedside, would supervise aides and housekeepers in the manner of foremen in a factory. For example, the bosses of Alta Bates Hospital in Berkeley, California, proposed changes that would slash the number of on-duty R.N.'s by 40%. Alta Bates even said the R.N.'s would have to apply and interview for their own jobs, held in some cases for as long as 20 years. Management's name for its scheme of reducing the professional attention given each patient is "patient-focused care."[134]

Although the single payer plan does not directly address the organization of health work, it brakes the financial interests driving toward the managed care model. Consequently, nurses and other hospital workers have been solid members of the single payer movement.

How Far Can Single Payer Reform Take Us?

The essence of the single payer plan is breaking the power of commercial health insurance corporations. This accomplishment is the basis for guaranteeing everyone the health care they need while putting a ceiling on costs. The average person would enjoy an improvement in health and in the treatment of ailments when they appear.

A single payer fund and its administration by an elected health commissioner will create an institution charged with continually improving the health of the population, giving it formidable means to realize the goal. This is a high point from which to deal with changes, but in political life new challenges always pop up.

Legal and administrative considerations necessarily limited the scope of the California Health Security Act, while threats to health arise from broad social forces. For example, imagine how a society not ruled by profit would deal with tobacco. Instead of slowly restricting cigarette companies decades after the menace of nicotine was proven, it would at a minimum immediately ban their advertising. The manufacture of one brand might be permitted, but the status game attached to a universe populated by cowboys and animated camels would be abolished. The number of sales outlets would be regulated, much as liquor stores are controlled, so that the addicted could get cigarettes with a little extra shopping effort. A single payer system, as a legal being, cannot do any of these things. Instead, it is left to deal with the medical legacy of the Marlboro man.

Health problems merge into larger social issues even more than the example of tobacco shows. Consider alcohol. Dependency on it in the late Soviet Union and Russia today is a symptom that work lost its social meaning as well as its role in supplying the means of life on a comfortable level (words that might apply to the problem of alcoholism here, too). The most progressive health commissioner might devote public health funds to combatting abuse of alcohol, tobacco, and drugs, but she could hardly solve the problem with the means available to her.

Nor can the single payer reform sweep away forever the simple quantitative issue of how much money to spend on health care. The payroll and individual income tax financing of the California Health

Security Act would keep the single payer fund at a fixed percentage of the gross domestic economy. The state legislature could change tax rates only by a two-thirds vote. This rule would provide stability for a few years at a time, and for workers a single payer plan is preferable to fragmented bargaining with companies to get health benefits through the job. However, pressures for adjustments would undoubtedly build in one way or another, just as they have in Germany, Sweden, and other countries.

Turning to economic relations within the health care industry, one point to note is that the single payer plan became relevant as insurance companies became the dominant power. Fifty years ago when independent physicians ruled medicine, conditions were hardly ripe for a single payer solution. Instead, the most far-reaching reform within the Western world was the solution found in the United Kingdom, nationalization of health care. Today, under a regime of corporatized medicine, people's anger is directed at the insurance companies, and the single payer banner reads, "Health care without insurance companies!"

The single payer movement had an opportunity, but may have been unable to grasp it, to slow down the centralization of capital. The California Health Security Act was officially neutral between physicians (and other health workers) organized in small practices reimbursed by a fee for service, and managed care organizations paid an annual capitation fee per enrollee. By being neutral, the Act might have halted the rush to managed care health plans. This is especially true for a superficial form of the latter. We may distinguish two kinds of plans: some HMOs have their own facilities and bring doctors into them, on salary or in partnerships of various sorts, to do the work of medicine at the HMO.

Plans of the second kind merely set themselves up between enrollees and a list of scattered physicians, labs, and other businesses, sometimes called "preferred providers". Preferred provider organizations (PPOs) are marketing schemes, gathering enrollees from employers as well as individually, then using their volume to negotiate discounts from independent health providers. A policy analyst for the California single payer campaign calls them "papier-maché" health plans.[135] If Proposition 186 had passed, its total freedom of choice for every cardholder, combined with uniform rates throughout the industry, would have wiped out most PPOs.

The moment for blocking the stampede into managed care plans may have passed. Once they get a big portion of the business, their market clout may be enough to compel most doctors to join them in order to get access to patients. The single payer movement must think about public insurance dealing with a health industry almost fully organized into managed care plans.

Furthermore, the technical and occupational forms of health care continue to change. The single payer plan deliberately interferes little with the spontaneous development of the forces of production in the industry. As the popular equation goes, single payer = private health care + public insurance. Industries develop as the result of different fragments of capital pursuing an anarchic search for higher profits. New big guys inevitably emerge. There are limits to the buying power of a health commissioner striving to get the best care for the least money from the owners of the means of production. Indeed, as seen in an earlier chapter when examining the United Kingdom, even public ownership cannot isolate an industry from the rest of the capitalist economy, from the pharmaceutical corporations, from suppliers eager for the right to get contracts from a national health service, etc.

Some leaders of the California movement, ignoring the fact that politics is the concentrated expression of economic relations, vowed great faith in the democratic operation of the single payer plan. They made several arguments:

1) The voters elect one person whom they judge on a single task: running the health security system. Unlike a governor, the health commissioner cannot divert public attention to other issues (immigration, crime, etc.).

2) The health commissioner is responsible for providing the benefits out of a fund whose size is set by law and whose appropriation process is automatic. The commissioner cannot point a finger of blame at other officials or at the legislature.

3) Politicians get their health care under the same system as everyone else, and just by being concerned about themselves they look

out for all cardholders. This happens because all but one in a thousand doctors will join the system (they must be in it or out), so that even wealthy and elite patients will get their care within the system.[136]

These are good arguments of pure civics. They put the case for one elected commissioner as opposed to an appointed board of neglectful, quarreling directors. However, anyone who reads the California Health Security Act can see that the commissioner has ways to carry out the job with more or less vigorous dedication.

More important, a view confined to civics fails to see that as economic forces develop and gather, they eventually change public institutions. This is not an argument against adopting a single payer plan. It is a warning that people must be aware of the limits of an institutional reform. Continued vigilance is required from a thriving single payer movement, which at its best is part of a larger people's movement. Just as capital is never satisfied with what it has, the people must know that capitalism forces them to struggle without sure foundation through one battle to the next.

A single payer plan would carry out a major overhaul of health insurance. This achievement, huge in itself, would leave problems in health care. It would not stop the march of events and trends. All in all, however, it would put the insurance corporations on the defensive and carry us down a new road toward the goal of all-round health as a normal state of being for everyone.

7

Big Capital Defeats Proposition 186

By summer 1993, people watching health reform could see that neither the Clintons nor a strong enough force in Congress would fight
for a single payer plan. For years progressive reformers had studied the
Canadian system and lobbied for single payer legislation. Now their
efforts flowed into the same stream as national politics.

A large California coalition of organizations, Health Access, had
pushed state legislation. Attorney Steve Schear had written the first
draft of what became known as the Petris bill. He worked out a compromise between people who want the law to preserve medicine
delivered by a fee for service and those who promote health maintenance groups that treat an enrollee for an annual charge. The bill
simply let both forms of medicine compete in the marketplace. The
largest audiences in memory who gathered for hearings in Sacramento
demanded that the legislature enact the Petris bill. By 1992 both hous-
es of the California legislature voted for it, but only by a majority. As a
money measure, the bill required a two-thirds vote to become law and
could not get it.

Late in 1992 a husband and wife pair of physicians, Vishu
Lingappa and Krista Farey, rewrote the Petris bill into an ideal single
payer plan, as much to clarify their thinking as for any other motive.
They changed the top authority from a commission appointed by the
governor, the House speaker, and so on to one commissioner elected by
the voters. California Physicians Alliance, a group in support of single
payer, took the Lingappa-Farey ideal seriously and put it through several rounds of criticism and rewrite.

In April 1993, Health Access appointed its annual subcommittee
to ponder an initiative. This year things got serious. Glen Schneider, a
health reformer with both Health Access and Neighbor to Neighbor,

joined Dr. Lingappa and Howard Owens, president of the Congress of California Seniors, a legislative advocacy coalition of 400 groups with 600,000 members. Beginning with text worked out by Lingappa and the doctors, this trio circulated, revised and remailed drafts. During the summer of 1993 they found Karl Manheim, a law professor who had worked on an initiative that rolled back automobile insurance rates. He and fellow attorneys helped rewrite the legislation so that it would repel challenges by the insurance companies.

Some people bowed to the lure of lobbying the Clinton or Mitchell plans in a more progressive direction. However, they were a minority, and enthusiasm built for launching a drive in 1994, even though everyone knew time would be short. As a practical organizer, Glen Schneider proposed a goal of raising $250,000 in pledges by the end of November 1993, with checkpoints along the way. Drs. Lingappa and Farey asked their colleagues at the California Physicians Alliance for $500 per member; a meeting pledged $25,000. Similar gifts from lawyers, teachers, and other individuals, with no big donations by any organization or wealthy person, reached the goal. Californians for Health Security (CHS) was born. In January 1994 it launched a 100-day signature drive.[137]

At the core of the CHS coalition are doctors opposed to corporatized medicine, senior citizens, and health reformers. Nurses and other health workers signed on early, as did political radicals who recognized the key struggle of 1994, and a number of trade unions, especially in service industries.

The organizational power behind the CHS campaign is Neighbor to Neighbor (N2N). Its executive director, Fred Ross, Jr., writes, "Most of the founding organizers of Neighbor to Neighbor were veterans of the United Farmworkers or were trained by my dad."[138] Fred Ross, Sr., arrived in California in 1952 and met Cesar Chavez. Together they carried out Ross's dream of founding Community Service Organizations along lines suggested by Saul Alinsky. He was a social theorist and activist who developed tactics notable for combining a lively, in-your-face spirit with mildly reformist purposes. His thinking follows the pragmatism of John Dewey and Robert Hutchins. N2N is a roving single issue group; at any one time it fights one major campaign, but it does not advocate a distinctive, long term social vision. When solidarity with Central American liberation struggles was its focus, N2N sponsored a boycott of Folger's coffee made with beans purchased from El Salvador's ruling elite. As that issue wound down, N2N turned to health reform. Organizers out of N2N were the backbone of the campaign waged by Californians for Health Security.

It is not easy to get 677,000 valid signatures, even in a state with a total of 22 million registered and potential voters. Most initiatives qualify for a statewide vote because a special interest pays signature gatherers. They basically pester folks at supermarkets, on campuses, and at other public locations. Perhaps a new low in the process occurred just when the single payer movement was being born. Philip Morris, Inc., and other tobacco companies qualified a measure by hiring canvassers who told prospective signers that it would regulate cigarettes when in fact it sought to overturn 300 local tobacco ordinances and nullify a state law.

Californians for Health Security filed 1,064,000 signatures on April 26, 1994, of which over 725,000 were valid. The country's first single payer voter referendum qualified for the Nov. 8, 1994 ballot. It aroused the soldiers of a new movement. CHS counts 10,000 canvassers who circulated petitions. Several people who were retired or who took leave from work gathered 5,000 signatures, and others obtained four, two, or one thousand signatures. Most volunteers signed up a few dozen to several hundred people on weekends. It is slogging work, measured at a rate of 15 to 30 signatures per hour. The gatherer announces the subject with a hook line over and over; discussions with people are only a distraction. In addition to circulators working on the street, labor unions collected signatures for the initiative through their organizational channels. Finally, CHS contracted with Voter Revolt, which is non-profit but hires canvassers. CHS paid Voter Revolt's expenses to gather 400,000 signatures.[139]

From the April deadline until the election season got under way after Labor Day, both sides prepared and fought their campaigns, although the struggle did not yet reach the public as a whole. An opposition coalition announced itself on May 26. Called Taxpayers Against the Government Takeover (TAGT), its member groups included the

Association of California Life Insurance Companies, a hospital association, the National Federation of Independent Businesses, and the state Chamber of Commerce.[140] Public filings would later show that 78% of its money came from insurance companies around the country.

The Campaign For Proposition 186

CHS campaign planners selected four key tools: 1) endorsements, 2) free media, 3) paid media, and 4) house parties. The course of events extended the list to six: CHS added a 5) visibility drive (stickers and signs) shortly before election day, and individuals and small teams of people carried out 6) spontaneous activities on their own.

Endorsements. Early in the summer CHS secured three important endorsements and began to gather hundreds more. A few senior citizens in CHS prodded the California unit of the American Association of Retired Persons to take a stand on the California Health Security Act. In June the AARP held four hearings around the state and endorsed the Act. The endorsement was a triumph for AARP members against the national headquarters, which never backed health care without insurance companies. The national office sells Medicare supplemental policies written by Prudential Insurance. In 1993 revenues from the operation provided over $100 million of AARP's $450 million total.

The League of Women Voters of California endorsed what was by July officially numbered Proposition 186. The League is sparing with its endorsements, making each one highly respectable. Besides seconding the usual arguments for a single payer plan, the League addressed some voters' concern about legislating in detail by initiative. The League noted, "A three year effort to reform the state's health care system through the legislative process failed.... Political reality is that we are very unlikely to achieve major reform of the health care system in the state or the nation unless the public takes the issue in its own hands."[141]

Through its west coast regional office, Consumers Union endorsed Proposition 186, too, as good news for both consumers of health care and doctors. A detailed five-page analysis supported a reform that makes obvious sense given plain vanilla liberal principles like progressive taxation. The statement did not shrink from saying that Consumers Union believes in "the elimination of insurers in the health care area."[142]

The endorsements by the AARP, LWV and CU, having five million members in California among them, gave Proposition 186 mainstream standing. Although TAGT would attack the measure with shrill, false labeling, it never raised the old cry that here is a communist plot to impose socialized medicine. Of course, a single payer plan is not socialized medicine, but since when has big capital respected facts? Instead, the three groups' support of the initiative probably helped TAGT realize that red-baiting would not work.

Almost 400 other groups and elected officials endorsed Proposition 186. The biggest category was 92 trade unions and labor federations, followed by church alliances, Democratic political clubs, city councils, ethnic organizations, and social service agencies. However, Democratic candidate for governor Kathleen Brown came out against the Act. The California Nurses Association put the most resources into its endorsement, mainly encouraging members to hold house parties.

CHS hired an organizer for the specific purpose of pushing campaign supporters to obtain small business endorsements, too. The idea was to blunt the opposition claim that business is united against a payroll tax that would allegedly cost jobs. Although 640 firms signed on to the resulting California Small Business Council, it never reversed the public's understanding that business opposed Proposition 186.

Free Media. Throughout the summer and the election season citizen spokespersons created a steady drumbeat of more than 50 op-ed pieces and dozens of letters to the editor, although the large circulation daily newspapers were most resistant. Advocates of Proposition 186 were speakers and panelists on over 300 talk shows, too.

Campaign supporters peppered the big dailies and the major television stations with demands to cover the proposition as vital news. Their thinking was that even biased coverage would stir interest as well as give grounds to reply with more opinion pieces. In August, CHS decided to spend $200,000 on a press relations operation designed to overwhelm the media and draw attention to Proposition 186 as the most significant decision on the ballot. Although the publicity campaign obtained much of the coverage just summarized, it did not compel the media to choose health reform as the main topic of the election. As we will see, the corporate media played their role in opposing Proposition 186.

In addition to media presentations, campaign speakers at 1,160 meetings of organizations, after-church talks, and other events reached more than 38,000 people with a detailed, first-hand message.

Paid media. CHS campaign planners decided that a paid television campaign was the key to victory. Polls they commissioned showed that voters divided into approximate thirds: in support of a single payer plan, firmly against it, and for it when they had enough information. "Most people get their information from TV."[143] Although CHS could not match the insurance industry dollar for dollar, the truth is on its side and it could win at least half the voters in the middle with television spots run in the last weeks before the election.

CHS set a goal of spending $1.2 million to $1.5 million on television. CHS leaders often voiced the sentiment that Proposition 186 would pass or fail based on whether the group could raise this amount of money. The logical conclusion was to funnel all efforts into this goal. As campaign manager Paul Milne noted, "You can do a little of a whole lot of things or you can do a whole lot of a couple of things."[144]

The ads began on Oct. 28 and ran twelve days until Nov. 8. CHS purchased $935,000 of television time, supplemented by a smaller amount spent on radio spots. Campaign volunteers funded the latter by telephoning supporters once again during the final month. The phone banking also used a national list of subscribers to the periodical *In These Times.*

House parties. The major tool for raising television money was house parties. Someone would host a party in her home, getting a dozen or more friends, coworkers, and neighbors to attend. A speaker from CHS would talk briefly, answer questions, then appeal for donations. From early summer to the last weekend before the election, CHS and Neighbor to Neighbor held 1,455 house parties that raised over one million dollars in individual donations of $25, $50 and $100. The drive set a record for a face-to-face method of raising money in a California political campaign. In addition, more than 22,000 attendees received detailed information about Proposition 186, obtained replies to questions they and their friends were asking, and were invited to become part of the campaign.

House parties did not just happen. The paid CHS staff was few in number, but nearly all organizers worked exclusively on house parties. They drove to a meeting with the host, then coached and coaxed her to send out at least 100 invitations which made it clear that the event was a fund raiser, not purely educational. They inquired every two or three days whether she was following up with telephone calls. The host asked people who could not attend to mail her a check for the campaign. The organizer attended parties, too, following the speaker's fund drive with an appeal for more people to hold their own house parties so that the process would continue.

Similarly, potential house party speakers prepared for and attended two or three training classes. In the early stages, organizers from Neighbor to Neighbor conducted the sessions. The instruction and role playing concentrated as much on the basic techniques of speaking (take a breath to collect yourself, establish your credentials, make eye contact, announce when you will answer two more questions, etc.) as on the script of the talk. The trial delivery of a potential speaker had to pass judgment. CHS assigned the best ones to house parties as top priority; others were more available to meet requests from clubs and organizations. The campaign staff convened a meeting of speakers every two or three weeks at which they brushed up on their role-playing and updated the message. House party speakers were on call to speak any evening and any time during the weekend. Arriving early to coordinate with the host and the organizer and leaving last, they gave three hours to each party. Many spoke three or four times a week for as many months. Certainly, people doing all sorts of work gave themselves fully to the campaign, but as a specialized unit, the house party speakers were the most devoted, unified, and highly trained volunteer cadre of CHS.[145]

Visibility kits. Although some bumper stickers were produced for the signature-gathering phase, most stickers and signs became available in the last two months. At first CHS sold them, but three weeks before Nov. 8 the organization urged people to take them for free and display them on cars and lawns in order to exhibit sentiment for Proposition 186 everywhere.

Spontaneous activities. People dedicated to single payer reform conducted many different activities either under the vague umbrella of CHS or on their own: demonstrations, fund raising entertainment events, raffles, debates, and, on the eve and dawn of the election, precinct walking. For example, the Gray Panthers of Berkeley with the League of Women Voters wrote and printed flyers, then distributed them at 7 a.m. to commuters at mass transit stops. An Alameda county subcommittee of Vote Health members made itself responsible for tabling at any public event where a crowd might be found. These people wrote and printed their own literature as much as they had official CHS supplies. The spontaneous activities were outside the main focus of television and fund raising for TV, and people carried them out without using money or paid organizers' time from CHS.

The Campaign Against Health Reform

Big capital applied ideological pressure through established channels of communication and opinion. The four main ones were paid television spots; employers' messages to employees; the corporate media, divided into news and editorial matter; and allegedly nonpartisan studies. The machinery already existed. Big capital did not need to build a movement, nor did it seriously try. Whatever else the campaign against Proposition 186 was, it was not a grass roots struggle. The servants of big capital held no demonstrations, conducted no house parties, and had no bumper stickers and lawn signs on the property of ordinary people (and few anywhere). Nearly all anti-186 spokespersons were hired guns instead of citizen volunteers. The closest that the opposition came to speech from below was in letters to the editor published in newspapers.

The message poured through official channels had a few basic themes. The two major ones were taxes and government. Capital told voters that Proposition 186 was a tax bill of $40 billion, the largest tax increase in California history, and people would be forced out of their private care and into government-run health care. Secondary themes raised the fear of hurting small business and losing 300,000 jobs while patients face rationing. Finally, like the owner of the sweatshop who goes to worship every weekend, most statements professed good intentions: we all want health reform that guarantees coverage everyone can afford, but Proposition 186 is the wrong way to do it. The right way remained a secret.

Big capital's anti-186 themes aroused doubt and cynicism about whether change is do-able, for the purpose of leading voters to vote No. The four established channels spoke with different tones, from alarmist to supposedly neutral, and they reinforced each other. Underlying the noise was the hint of a bully: big capital will not cooperate with this reform, so don't make a mess by trying.

The two major themes were lies in the form of half truths. Yes, Proposition 186 will raise taxes by $40 billion. It also saves $40 billion in insurance premiums, deductibles and copayments, and expenses out of pocket. Furthermore, 96% of the dollars will provide health care, while insurance companies deliver only $30 billion of care for the same amount of money.

As for government-run health care, a single payer fund intrudes less on doctors and other private providers than do insurance companies and managed care plans today. Once the ordinary citizen receives her health security card, she may never have contact with the state again. She simply visits the private clinic, HMO plan, or doctor's office of her choice. These providers, competing on quality, could actually improve their service once they are freed of the shackles of private insurers.

The notion that minor taxes on small business would discourage new ventures and even result in the loss of existing jobs is a repeat of the common reactionary argument that it is disastrous to raise the minimum wage, enact family leave legislation, and in any way hoist life up from conditions of slavery. Here the claim is that when every small restaurant, for example, must pay a 4.4% payroll tax, their simultaneous increase of menu prices by twenty-five cents would drive many of them out of business and handicap California in the global competition among Italian bistros. Experience with raising the minimum wage justifies a sarcastic appreciation of this line.

Even a spirited reply to big capital's themes concedes ground to them. None of the rebuttal just summarized lays out the advantages of a single payer plan over private health insurance. Advocates of single payer can be proud of an open (hence debate-filled) system compared to our total lack of input, influence, and power over the bosses of

Aetna, Prudential, and the other private insurers. A single payer fund is essential if we are going to make health care a right for everyone.

A twist in the anti-186 themes is that they actually build on the failures of…the commercial market. Today we suffer from a bureaucracy managed by insurance companies. Today we accept rationing of care according to the terms of our policy, if any, out of the endless variety of provisions written and sold in the market. Big capital's themes transfer the negative atmosphere to the solution. In order to accomplish this feat, they rely on a non-class outlook or at least on the view that government performs worse than corporate institutions. Big capital's hidden threat to wreck a single payer reform weighs in here, too. Although one can argue the points of fact and the sensible provisions of the single payer plan, the effective reply must be in the form of a movement of people that stands up to big capital and asserts that things are going to be different from now on.

Let us examine how capital used its various channels in mutual support of each other.

Paid television. Taxpayers Against the Government Takeover began television commercials before the traditional Labor Day election kickoff. They were a steady drumbeat of the lies already mentioned. Produced by Richard Wiebe's operation out of Los Angeles (the same firm that made the "Harry and Louise" commercials), the anti-186 spots used actors portraying small business owners, nurses, and just plain folks. Except for one spot lampooning the health commissioner, their tone was cooler than the negative ads run by candidates. They delivered their message, that Proposition 186 would be a disastrous mistake, firmly but without making it the big issue of the election. To achieve this goal, the ads ran for weeks and weeks but never flooded the airwaves.

Insurance companies and managed care plans paid the bill for television. TAGT collected $5.8 million by Sept. 30. The largest single gift was $1.6 million from the Health Insurance Association of America in Washington, D.C., whose members write about 25% of California's health insurance. The California Association of Hospitals and Health Systems donated the next largest amount, $409,681. Individual companies gave, too. Among them were the following:

Individual corporate donations against Prop. 186

Calif. Physicians Ins. Corp.	$355,000
PacifiCare of California	243,068
HealthNet	200,000
Aetna	190,923
Connecticut General	179,161
Prudential	169,661
Travelers	169,161
MetLife	164,161
Blue Cross	150,000
Foundation Health Plan	105,000
National Medical Enterprises	100,000

Insurance companies alone provided 78% of TAGT's funds. [146]

However, insurance companies know they have a bad image, so they hid behind others—by telling more lies. TAGT ads claimed that nurses and senior citizens oppose Proposition 186. As a list of groups rolled by at the end of their commercials, a viewer might catch the names of the Congress of Nursing Executives and The Seniors Coalition. The nurse executives' have 1,100 members who have left the bedside for top management, versus the California Nurses Association, whose 25,000 nurses supported Proposition 186 fervently and worked hard for it. TAGT literature claimed that The Seniors Coalition speaks for 325,000 Californians (one-tenth the three million in AARP's California chapter), but the shop is a direct mail operation in Virginia founded by super-conservative Richard Viguerie and convicted extortionist Dan Alexander.[147] The State of Maryland banned it from raising funds, and the State of Pennsylvania fined it.

TAGT admits to $4.9 million spent on television and radio, plus $2 million on direct mail. In addition, the campaign coincided with the annual open enrollment period during which many employees may change health plans obtained through work. The insurance companies seemed to spend more money than usual on advertising with a soft sell designed to make people feel good about their choices in the existing system of commercial insurance.

Employer messages. TAGT supplied employers with an example of a letter they could distribute to employees. Wells Fargo among other corporations devoted a column of its employee newsletter to opposing Proposition 186. The first of its seven reasons said, "The proposal would replace the choice of insurance plans that Wells Fargo employees currently enjoy with a one-size-fits-all package of government-approved benefits."[148] A worker might be tempted to reply: yes, equality for everyone and comprehensive health care as a right, including all doctor and hospital bills as well as long term care, plus more, guaranteed with no deductibles, no maximum payout, and one small copayment ($5 for a prescriptions filled outside a hospital or doctor's office)—that one size would fit me just fine.

It is only a temptation to reply like that. Democracy in a capitalist society stops at the entrance to the workplace. Every worker knows that it is not a good idea to oppose the company in front of more than a few trusted coworkers, not by initiating discussion and even less by handing out a printed leaflet in reply. (This rule applies to the individual; it collapses when a mass movement provides safety in numbers.) Ambitious employees at middle and higher levels take the cue to speak up in agreement with the employer. The worker's need to be cautious, even furtive, with her opinion instills pessimism about whether Proposition 186 can pass. Each isolated supporter sees the powers that be dominating the public stage with misinformation.

A related channel for the insurance companies was their agents. Some of them proved they were eager beavers by writing letters to policy holders.

Academic studies. TAGT's commercials were the openly partisan channel for big capital's message. The most hidden were two policy studies by allegedly neutral parties. In August 1994 the Institute for Governmental Studies at the University of California published the most used one, written by Dwayne Banks. His main point was a claim that the California Health Security Act is not adequately financed and would face a revenue shortfall starting at $13 billion in 1996 and growing rapidly in succeeding years. The gap would compel rationing or higher taxes.

Banks confirmed the opinion that professors are available to be servants of the "hire learning." Under immediate and massive criticism from policy analysts who favor a single payer plan, he admitted to \$11 billion of miscalculations and simple errors of addition, but he and his masters stuck by his conclusions. If one wanted to wage a war of policy studies, expert opinion universally admitted that single payer saves money compared to the existing marketplace and compared to every other alternative. The Congressional Budget Office and the General Accounting Office said so. Dorothy Rice, once the federal government's top health statistician, reviewed the analysis of costs and revenues behind Proposition 186 and wrote that it "is carefully formulated and fiscally sound." At a state senate hearing on Sept. 9, she testified that Banks's study is entirely wrong.[149]

Intellectuals supporting Proposition 186 attended the press conference at which the Institute for Governmental Studies released Banks's fiction, handing out proof that Dwayne Banks can't add. It did not matter. Big capital's media had what they needed. Banks's paper became an unquestioned study when the *San Francisco Chronicle* wrote its editorial against Proposition 186.[150] The supposedly neutral Legislative Analyst, writing in the pamphlet mailed to every voter, used Banks's figures. (In his report the Analyst added several factual errors of his own.)

The other major study used by big capital originated with the Kaiser Family Foundation, which has no formal connection with the Kaiser plan. On Oct. 26 it released a report written by the accounting firm KMPG Peat Marwick. The document admitted that the single payer plan would reduce administrative costs for health care by \$9 billion a year, that on average individuals would save \$550 a year, and that business would save \$2 billion a year (although some companies would gain while others paid their share for the first time). However, by ignoring the cost-saving elements of single payer and assuming that medical inflation would continue at 8% a year rather than the 5% used by policy analysts evaluating single payer plans, the accountants gave corporate media their headline: "Study Says Prop. 186 Would Swell Deficit."[151] The newspaper reported Kaiser's "independent study" and recalled Banks's "independent analysis."

The partisan nature of the Kaiser paper was shown by the timing of its release. The foundation was on top of an issue that had brewed for months in its field of specialty. Yet somehow it could not get out a report until less than two weeks before election day. Banks's tale provided the early ammunition, while Kaiser sprang a clincher too late for serious rebuttal. Furthermore, the foundation apparently did not protest the media's one-sided use of its report. Immediately after the election, a foundation officer repeated big capital's anti-186 themes: "Voters are saying no to new taxes and no to big government."[152]

Late in the summer the Chamber of Commerce, which opposed Proposition 186, agreed to host a series of debates around the state. The pro-initiative side won the first two of them. This experience is general throughout the country: when both sides talk at reasonable length to any audience of ordinary people, they favor the single payer solution. The Chamber canceled or evaded the rest of the agreed debates. So-called balanced academic studies are great, but genuine forums have no place in the arsenal of misrepresentation.

Media. Between openly partisan paid television and phony balanced studies were the corporate media. Their first decision was how much coverage Proposition 186 needed. The daily press and television have considerable power to set a public agenda, as shown by their occasional crusades to right a minor wrong. Until late September the media gave single payer health reform practically no coverage. Then they presented some debate, using their tools to tilt it. These include one-sided headlines, like the one for the Kaiser study quoted above, and an air of neutrality between opposing studies, even when one side was clearly incorrect. Television created confusion (and therefore gave pause about adopting a change) with a rush of quick, incoherent sound bites. Supposedly more thoughtful media, like the MacNeil/Lehrer News Hour, ran a two-to-one format: voices for, those against, and a falsely neutral commentator like the head of the Kaiser Foundation.

The media strayed into editorializing in the news, too. For example, a reporter doing a story on cutbacks and management turmoil at California Pacific Medical Center concluded with a general paragraph on the alleged incentive for plans that collect a per-enrollee fee to keep their members healthy.[153] As we have seen, managed care plans do not come close to preventive health detection and treatment and in fact have a short term outlook.

In labeled editorials the corporate media acted as though they were not part of big capital. "To say that changes are needed in a state where 6 million are uninsured is to say the obvious." Then the editorial writer cited a phony study, worried about job loss, repeated the half-truth that taxes will rise (while not mentioning the insurance companies once), and wrung his hands over a commissioner described as a health czar because she would have a fraction of the power that insurance company chiefs possess today.[154]

A few hundred CHS volunteers lobbied the media intensely for full and fair treatment of the major public issues raised by Proposition 186. They had only marginal effect. The press knew that the single payer movement had involved several tens of thousands of people. On the other hand, 100,000 people in southern California marched against Proposition 187, and big capital split on whether attacking immigrants was a good idea. After these events the mass media scrambled to get on board before the train left the station and to maintain the appearance of covering the immigration debate.

Do the mass media follow public opinion or make it? Corporate-owned media followed capital's overall stand in opposition to a single payer plan. Major daily newspapers and television stations did so not merely because insurance companies and managed care plans advertise with them, but also and more fundamentally because these entertainment and news outlets are a section of big capital, indeed, one of its most politicized and class conscious parts.

Outcome of the Campaign

According to the Field poll for California, most voters did not hear about Proposition 186 until late in the campaign season. In July, the poll found 16% against, 13% for, 9% undecided, and 62% did not know about it. By mid-September, the results were 28% against, 20% for, 10% undecided, and 42% still not aware of the issue.[155]

Among opinion tallies, the most favorable report ever made public came in September from the Kaiser Family Foundation. It found voters going 38% for Proposition 186, 34% against, and 28% undecided. Because of variations in the wording of questions and subtle aspects of polltakers' behavior, surveys from different organizations are not comparable.

On election eve and the day itself, single payer recruits helped the Democratic Party to get out the vote. They hung slate cards on the doors of homes where a favorable vote was likely. This effort occurred in selected areas, like Berkeley and Oakland in northern California.

Results on Nov. 8 showed that the single payer movement had filled the glass one-quarter full. Two million Californians, just under 27%, voted for Proposition 186. The people of San Francisco voted 55% in favor of it, as did Oakland voters. Berkeley went almost three to one for the initiative. In Alameda County, which combines the cities of Oakland and Berkeley with more conservative areas in the east and south, 40% voted for Proposition 186.

In part, the vote is a result of forces beyond control once a campaign was launched. The time from January to November, during which CHS carried out both a signature drive and a completely new issue campaign, was short. In addition, the entire surrounding political climate was difficult. Although pundits say the voters were angry at government, they seemed rather to be disgusted with President Clinton and New Democrats. They are the ones who lost seats in Congress, while most sponsors of the McDermott single payer bill did not, and no member of the Congressional Black Caucus was defeated. Voters did toss aside New Democrats, especially in the South, and they turned to conservative Republicans to replace them. The left wing of the Democratic Party, if the term has a meaning these days, held most of its seats, but it certainly made no advances. In this atmosphere the charges of more government and more taxes against Proposition 186 had their effect.

Big capital defeated Proposition 186. Listening to the most active volunteers as tallies came in Nov. 8, this writer found two reactions. One was a sentiment of no regrets, indeed a feeling of deep satisfaction, that they had waged a campaign, rushed as it was and in a difficult year. Without it, the main thing everyone would say about health reform is that it failed in Washington and has even less chance in the next Congress. Because of Proposition 186 that is not the case. A spokesperson for a national lobbying group for single payer said four days after the election, "California kept health reform alive."[156] Within the state, thousands of people got involved, learned the issue, and made a commitment. They are the base of future struggles. Instead of being a spectator to the dreary national scene, instead of confining oneself to making requests on the Clinton administration and Democratic office-holders, activists have started down the road toward arousing the people to demand their right of health care.

The second attitude was a desire to learn. Proposition 186 lost badly, and handicaps like too little time and the political atmosphere of the year do not explain the low figure of less than 27%. Furthermore, Californians for Health Security carried out a strategy in pure form. Energetic, selfless campaign workers gave the game plan the best possible test. For anyone who has worked in progressive coalitions, CHS was remarkable for the absence of divisions and contention, endless or otherwise. However, people were thinking. They noted events like scientists observing an experiment. It is time to review the campaign to figure out what went well and what CHS or its counterparts in other states must do differently in order to win.

8

Build a Movement or Sell a Product?

Proposition 186 lost on election day, but the campaign for it gave us some positive lessons.

One was house parties. They are an excellent channel for taking a message to a dozen or more generally favorable people, answering their specific questions, and then persuading them to join the campaign. House parties demand work. An organizer who stays in touch with the host and encourages her to keep reaching out and getting back to attendees is crucial. The host herself must examine her position in society to find coworkers, friends, members of social group or church, and neighbors who are open to the reform. A speaker must know the campaign's political message as well as details of the single payer plan, blending the two in favor of basic politics. She must pursue a goal, which is to draw the inescapable connection that runs from a good idea to personal action.

Although Californians for Health Security (CHS), the coalition for Proposition 186, aimed house parties at raising money, they can arouse people to political deeds, from writing a customized leaflet for one's workplace to canvassing a precinct. As run by CHS, house parties enjoyed a good return for a fund raising operation. It cost $330,000 in paid organizer time and overhead expenses to raise almost $1 million. Ironically, a more directly political use of house parties would accept a lower ratio of revenue to expense. Certainly, the house party machine would aim to be self-supporting financially and raise money for the campaign, too. However, it would appeal more for new recruits and urge them to join various activities. Directing house parties to this end would allow, even require, that they be held among all the different communities of working people.

A second lesson of the campaign was that the big political picture wins support, not the clever marvels of policy. As one house party speaker wrote after the election, "It is important for single-payer advocates to be fluent about the single-payer concept and on specific provisions of the initiative.... However, successful organizing efforts challenged and inspired people with the campaign's political message: Take power away from insurance corporations and give it back to the people. Stop the insane waste in human health and human lives. Invest in each other's (and our children's) health. Guarantee everyone protection from being impoverished by health care costs."[157]

Steve Schear, chair of the advocacy group Vote Health, often made the point that we must compare Proposition 186 not with some perfect ideal but with the alternative, that is, the disaster created by a market of commercial insurance. When Quentin Young, M.D., a founder of Physicians for a National Health Plan, spoke during a trip to California in August 1994, he put the question squarely: you are voting on whether the insurance companies and managed care plans will become the robber barons of the 21st century or whether we will establish that health care is a right.[158]

Third, big capital could not dismiss the single payer plan as the dream of a fringe group, because CHS nailed down several key endorsements. The American Association of Retired Persons in California, the League of Women Voters, and Consumers Union endorsed Proposition 186. The insurance companies never dared to suggest that these groups were dupes of radicals promoting socialized medicine.

Fourth, the California campaign proved that the right to health care is an idea whose time has come. Several thousand people gave their lives to it. They worked hard for almost a year. The volunteers did not fit one mold. Although they were mostly white and college educated, some had been politically active for years while others were in their first campaign. Their average age was higher than the general population, but they were young, middle aged and old. A voice inside each of them said, "This thing is about more than health reform, important as that is. What are we doing in our lives that is more urgent than helping this movement take a step forward?"

Since, however, California did not have a single payer plan the morning after Nov. 8, people must figure out what needs to change. CHS held two long days of meetings after the election to begin the job. Although votes were not taken, nearly everyone would agree on a few conclusions, like involving and reaching all elements of the working people instead of being a group of educated white persons. Supplies of literature must be available earlier and in sufficient quantity. In a large state like California, a campaign must solve the problem of coordinating activity and allocating resources between the San Francisco Bay Area, which enjoys a dense network of organizations that started the whole thing, and the less organized, sprawling, and massively populated southland. With more time, like the two years now available before another initiative might be mounted, there should be more consultation with potential allies to work out details. For example, California retirees who might choose to move out of state have concerns that should and can be addressed.

Beyond these shortcomings, campaigners drew a number of lessons that add up to the choice put in the title of this chapter: are we building a movement or selling a product? The direction, strategy, and essential action of CHS amounted to doing the latter. The result was a big loss, a 73% vote against Proposition 186. The following lessons taken one by one might seem obvious, but CHS showed that it is possible to act in a contrary manner and suffer the consequences.

Lesson 1: Decide who will make health reform happen

Obviously, the insurance companies oppose reform. Is the single payer plan in the fundamental interest of everyone else? No, in this social question as in most others, the interests of classes are opposed. Those who benefit most from a single payer plan (people without health coverage, employees with tattered and constricting coverage through the employer, senior citizens on fixed income, etc.) are sections of the working people. On the other hand, big capital in general will never be happy about making health care a right. Small business is divided and not a major force for reform. A previous chapter argued in detail about class interests.

CHS hired a staff person who prompted volunteers to get business endorsements of Proposition 186. CHS did not devote similar resources to energizing workers. Trade unions in the service sector gave money to CHS. The California Nurses Association, and to a lesser degree the International Longshoremen and Warehousemen's Union, promoted fund raising house parties by their members. CHS did not go back in the opposite direction, that is, it did not build a movement among workers, neither through trade unions where appropriate nor by opening new channels. There was a San Francisco labor committee for single payer, but it was a minor footnote of the campaign.

After the Nov. 8 defeat, some CHS leaders talked about concessions in the single payer law itself. For example, instead of an elected commissioner, the California Health Security Act could specify an appointed commission, with a couple of seats reserved for business (employers), one for hospitals, a seat to physicians, one to health maintenance organizations, etc. This arrangement would sell off chunks of power in hope of getting support for enacting the reform. Similarly, the last shred of progressive taxation of income, the surcharge on income above $250,000 per person, could be eliminated in the hope of attracting financial support for a campaign from big money in Hollywood or elsewhere.

Strategists mull over concessions because they assume one way or another that they, a handful of far-seeing social policy analysts, must sell the single payer plan to the capitalist class. It in turn will nudge moderate and conservative voters our way. While aware that the insurance companies are the enemy, this outlook appeals to other centers of money and established power. The result is an attempt at selling health reform to capital on practical business terms.

When the California coalition Health Access wrote bills for the state legislature in the early 1990s, they became ensnared in bargaining with special interests like the hospitals. Health Access made concessions at the request of the hospital association, and then the latter did not endorse the bill anyway.[159]

The opposite choice looks at who has won big changes previously, and how they did it. The working class won the eight-hour day. Working people caused the reforms of the New Deal. Social Security happened not because Franklin D. Roosevelt was a generous man but because masses fought for it. The 1960s civil rights and black power movements were struggles of the people, and Lyndon Johnson merely responded to them. On the same principle but on the reverse side of the coin, Johnson obeyed big capital instead of the masses on Vietnam, and he went down. His personal defeat was a by-product of the movement that was essential to stopping U.S. aggression in Indochina. The movement for the right to health care follows this proud history, if its strategists can answer the fundamental question of which classes will make health reform happen.

Activists who want to rely on the working people would modify the single payer plan in the opposite direction from those who hope that concessions will buy the assent of capital. For example, they say get rid of the individual income tax on most people and collect a progressive tax on high incomes. As it is, the personal income tax raises only 10% of the single payer fund. Let's finance the system mostly or even totally with employer-based levies.

Whom must we rely on, big capital or the working class? This question was also the basic choice underneath the controversy about so-called illegal immigrants and their health rights. As explained in a previous chapter, the California Health Security Act left the rules open to future legislatures. However, the leaders of CHS specified the decision in advance by writing in the State-mailed voter's guide that benefits would go only to legal California residents. Why? Number-watchers' early polls told them that if voters hear that illegal immigrants get public health care, Proposition 186 loses.

Yet opposition to the anti-immigrant Proposition 187 grew from 20% in surveys to 41% of the final ballot, while Proposition 186 declined from its best poll showings to less than 27% of the vote. The result was that single payer lagged behind immigrant defense by 14 points. In liberal Alameda County, where voters actually rejected Proposition 187, the gap was wider, a lag of 20 points.[160] CHS catered to the racism of conservative voters, but big capital crushed the single payer health plan anyway. CHS strategists achieved both loss of principles and greater defeat because they were confused about which class to rely on.

Lesson 2: Appeal to collective interest
CHS's literature and standard speech went directly to individual cal-

culation and kept it isolated from collective interest. In response to polls and focus groups, the campaign strategists were proud of literature that began with an invitation to "Take the Health Security Test" and see how you are at risk. A quiz asked eight questions, beginning, "Does your health insurance pay for long-term care at home or in a nursing home?" Then the leaflet or speech presented the single payer plan as a sound, workable solution.

Certainly, everyone calculates how she will fare under a reform. However, the relevant opposite of self-interest is not altruism or self-denial (this is not a drive to recruit monks and nuns) but collective interest. For example, a movement must ask the individual, are you one of the so-many millions of workers who would lose your health care if you lost or even changed your job? Collective interest exists because the individual can obtain something only when the people as a whole get it. Every movement based on working people reminds them of this fact, and they respond to its truth, whether the demand is for unemployment insurance, public education, or health insurance.

CHS's individualistic approach betrayed the hand of the advertiser selling a product. Ad men think they know what moves people—greed and fear. You must appeal to one, the other, or both. In fact, CHS's planners relied on an advertising genius and a political consultant, and the result was to sell a product instead of building a movement. Unfortunately for these experts, voters were asked to approve the launch of a new company, the Health Security System, and commit to buying its product. After the vote went against it, most individuals pass on to their next consumer decision. But when a movement loses a battle, everyone in it knows that "they" (big capital) denied millions of people their right. With good leadership, a movement regroups and fights on until victory.

By showing persons that they are part of a mass of people being denied what is theirs, a movement taps motives that inspire working people: doing the right thing, and doing it arm in arm with sisters and brothers.

Lesson 3: Drive home a slogan and a noun phrase
CHS never focused people on the principle, "Health care is a right!"

The campaign did not have a main slogan. Perhaps the closest it came was the individualistic tag line, "Get the health security you're already paying for." A movement needs a slogan, but if one is selling a product, a variety of cute lines will do, like, "Prop. 186. It's Good for Everyone."

Similarly, a movement needs a noun phrase to summarize the distinct essence of its goal. CHS shied away from "single payer plan," perhaps because people thought it was a technical term that only an in-group understands. That may be the case. However, CHS never chose a meaningful substitute. The term in its name, in the Act, and in much literature was "health security." The phrase is too ambiguous for use by a movement. President Clinton is for health security and apple pie. Imagine that someone in our movement asks a friend at work, "What do you think of Proposition 186?" The friend shoots back, "What's that?" Our activist needs a handy answer, for example, "Health care without insurance companies." A noun phrase is vital to concentrate and distinguish the movement's goal.

A slogan and a noun phrase help a movement to express a collective, public, and social demand. They raise the benefits of the solution to the level of principle. They draw a line between our side and the enemy. The ad man, in contrast, wants a quick decision to buy, which he seeks to win by stating individual benefits with cute mottos. For him, the connection between consumer and us is simply a positive glow around the name of our brand, Proposition 186. If a campaign is selling a product, it can get by with a variety of clever ad lines that most people are too embarrassed to use in ordinary speech.

Part of the reason why CHS did not rally around a slogan and a noun phrase goes back to the decision of who will fight for health reform. At the Alameda County kickoff rally on Sept. 11, 1994, the moderator counseled that campaign supporters avoid the term "universal coverage" because some people get the impression from it that they would pay for a free ride by others (that is, poor people). Like a dozen other misconceptions, the campaign had to decide whether to tell people the actual story or to abandon every distinctive phrase and evade questions. In this case, the reply is that because of cost shifting in the health industry, people already pay for others through higher premiums. How much can we finesse our way past erroneous attitudes?

Which ideological questions must we engage instead of avoiding? Can we find and arouse people to our side precisely because we show them how big capital misleads them?

Lesson 4: Don't fight in TV alley

CHS put in writing the assumption that underlay its entire campaign strategy. A document for potential speakers at house parties said, "If we all contribute as much as we can and are willing to ask others to do the same, we can launch our own paid media campaign and beat the opposition at their own game."[161] The specific paid medium was television. As the standard speech had it, "Most people get their information from TV."[162]

Consequently, the campaign for Proposition 186 was largely a fund raising drive for television. As a result, so much else that should have been done was not done. House party speakers aimed to get the maximum donation from each party for the television buy. Something like 85% of paid staff time was devoted to raising money for television, counting the house party operation in this category. Volunteers could form committees to do anything, like hold small demonstrations and get out to crowds and events on weekends, but they were scattered and had no substantial resources to build such activities. In fact, volunteers for a long time had no official literature or scarce amounts of it. First, the money was set aside for television. Second, the consultants and strategists took weeks to conduct research and refine the vital television message, so they had no time to rush out literature.

The plan involved buying media time from election day backwards, because most people make up their minds just before they vote. Enormous tension built up in the campaign by keying everything to the television spots that would debut eventually. The best thing one could do was raise money for them. Attendees at house parties were asked to give for the television ads to come. Opinion surveys that showed Proposition 186 losing were "already outdated" because "none of the polls taken so far…measure the impact of our ad campaign," said a CHS statement dated Oct. 27.[163]

Although the insurance companies could buy as many millions of dollars of attack ads as they wished, campaign planners still committed to fighting in TV alley. The truth is on our side, so CHS did not need to match the insurance companies dollar for dollar. We had an advertising agency (Hal Larson) with a brilliant no-loss record of political television. Back in 1988, voters approved Proposition 103, a rollback of automobile insurance rates, despite a $70 million campaign by the insurance companies. So they were caught by a dilemma: dump in as much money and suffer the same counterproductive backlash, or spend less and lose to our brilliant spots. As it happened, the CHS-hired political consultant, Bill Zimmerman, had spent $1.5 million in 1988 running the successful campaign for Proposition 103.

During the summer, leading CHS officials voiced the opinion that Proposition 186 would pass or fail depending on whether we could spend $1.5 million on television. However, in the second week of September, the ad guru, Hal Larson, told campaign manager Paul Milne that Proposition 186 would pass if he could spend $2.7 million.[164] It would be overly cynical to conclude that one man pulled a monstrous bait-and-switch tactic on CHS. The campaign manager and his colleagues accepted the approach of fashioning a media drive that would sell the product. The earliest organizations to give major donations were the California Teachers Association and the Service Employees International Union. They agreed to a professional political campaign and specifically marked five-figure gifts for polls and focus groups to assess if and how such a campaign would win.

In the end, CHS raised just over a million dollars for television and radio. This amount paid to produce and run for twelve days two 30-second television spots. One consisted of several quick endorsement statements by representatives of major groups like the AARP. The other, praised before release by CHS's organization director for memorable pictures, made an emotional appeal to give our children health security. If one believes opinion polls, and allowing for their margin of error, the television campaign reduced the vote against Proposition 186 by zero to four percent.

Lesson 5: Invest in educating people

A movement must build commitment in people. Commitment is a product of felt needs and reflection. According to some views, human emotion is like animal affect, at war with reason and barely tamed by external or internal constraint. Progressive movements belie this opinion and demonstrate that the strongest, deepest, and most self-sacrificing attachments among people are the product of reason. In the history of our species, thinking arises with labor, the activity which distinguishes us from animals. Emotion and human commitments are formed by labor and thought. Take the example of Bartolomeo Vanzetti, a self-taught worker framed with Nicola Sacco after they dared to protest the death of an immigrant in federal custody. Abstract principles made solid over a lifetime are at one with Vanzetti's defiant acceptance of a death sentence:

> "If it had not been for this thing, I might have live out my life talking at street corners to scorning men. I might have die, unmarked, unknown, a failure. Now we are not a failure. This is our career and our triumph. Never in our full life can we hope to do such work for tolerance, for justice, for man's understanding of man, as now we do by an accident. Our words,—our lives—our pains—nothing! The taking of our lives—lives of a good shoe maker and a poor fish peddler—all! That last moment belong to us—that agony is our triumph!"[165]

CHS volunteers and paid staff produced a large number of educational items. The problem is that the center of the campaign used none of it in a mass way. As noted above, the television strategy delayed the production of the main leaflets and brochures. When they appeared, activists immediately noted that they were difficult to photocopy. The official leaflets were on expensive coated paper, off-white with blue headlines and gray halftone backgrounds. At first, people who wanted bulk quantities were asked to purchase them at ten cents a piece. In October CHS published a photocopiable but still two-sided sheet on ordinary bond stock, but it was always in short supply. CHS never had mass quantities of a cheap, one-page leaflet. At least one supporter produced on her own a few thousand copies of a four-page tabloid in newspaper format, but she did not have channels of distribution to take them all.

The organization spent $125,000 on printed materials, including items designed to make the campaign visible (bumper stickers and window signs) rather than to educate. This is one-eighth of the television and radio expenditure. In 30- and 60-second spots, television cannot educate. At two cents per copy of a cheap leaflet, $200,000 would buy ten million copies. It would be necessary to spend a little more, too, for paid organizers to coordinate distribution by volunteers. This effort would have diverted momentum from the house parties, the core of fund raising for television. In fact, the house party program would have changed, asking attendees to join the campaign as leafleters, diluting the appeal to make all one's sacrifice through one's checkbook.

Patient education is especially important when the issue is single payer health reform. Any CHS worker can testify that it takes time to persuade people that here is a step we must take. Unlike so many referendums that pose a reactionary cutback or denial of human rights, Proposition 186 was a constructive step forward. However, people want to be sure about the consequences before they agree to it. The payoff for education is that once convinced, people do not merely nod assent. They become solid, fervent supporters of single payer health care.

Lesson 6: Agitate, get feedback, agitate

When a campaign decides to publish leaflets by the millions, it does not print them all at once. Instead, it should produce and distribute moderate quantities of an item and seek feedback from people. CHS chose a different method using the tools of those who sell a product: focus groups and opinion polls. Perhaps these tools work in a competition between cola corporations or between mainstream politicians, when choice A is only marginally different from choice B.

Opinion polls discourage the respondent from regarding herself as a participant in a movement. They lead her to react like an individual consumer or a voter in the polling booth. The survey encourages a passive attitude. The polled person tells the research organization what she thinks, and they take it from there; she only indicates how she would vote if the election were held today. The format of questions posed by a stiff-mannered poll taker and answers framed as a multiple choice or fill-in-the-blank is a world apart from a political dialogue with an acquaintance or coworker.

Focus groups told strategists that health consumers respond to themes like security, choice, and affordability. However, when CHS representatives spoke at meetings and to people on the street, the key discussions did not go along lines of individualistic consumerism. Some people supported Proposition 186 because they believe in the right to health care or in the value of a social investment in it. Persons who have no social vision were typically not enthusiastic no matter how much the initiative might save them personally. They were sceptical that the plan could work, and capital's slogans against government had an effect on them.

CHS's campaign director Paul Milne believes in polls and focus groups. After Nov. 8 he told their story. A year ago, a poll showed that 40% had a negative feeling toward the insurance companies and 40% had a negative attitude toward government. The strategy therefore was for paid media to take single payer health reform from 40% to 50% plus one vote. But by mid-summer 1994, 60% had a negative attitude toward government while hostility toward insurance companies remained at 40%. The quandary then, he implied, was to persist with the strategy and hope that television would perform a miracle, or somehow to change course.

The problem for the number-watcher is that an opinion poll is a shallow sampling at one moment. Polls are not a tool of a science of history; they do not reveal how the struggle between classes will play out. In order to gain any insight and therefore foresight about the latter, people must engage in the practice of building a movement. By taking action and enrolling others to take action, a movement learns the real currents of social development and where they might flow. However, the lures of consumerist politics seduced CHS leaders into relying on polls to investigate the world and television to change it.

Lesson 7: Grab the moment for a march

A coalition like CHS cannot by itself create a mass march and rally. However, a movement always looks for signs that a large demonstration could happen. It might be done through organizations that are willing and able to get their members out, or it might tap the sentiment of tens of thousands of people more spontaneously, as defenders of immigrants found when 100,000 marched against Proposition 187.

A big march gives a boost to the participants, and the feeling spreads far beyond them. The movement's slogan on banner after banner gets new respect. Although the gains from a rally do not depend on the corporate media, it gives them a tough choice: convey the event and its scope reasonably honestly and thereby enlarge its impact, or under-report it and lose credibility with the tens of thousands of people who were there.

Some activists felt that the campaign did not pay attention to smaller protests and direct action. Sometimes CHS did consider them, but strategists evaluated opportunities exclusively on the criteria of whether the media would report them and how they would look on television, not whether the event would dampen spirits or intensify the desire to organize bigger rallies.

Lesson 8: Build through group and personal channels

The house parties followed this lesson to multiply themselves. Friends and coworkers of the host who attended her party were the source of hosts for the next round of parties. Otherwise, the campaign played down opportunities that did not flow directly into raising funds for television.

One worker at a large company can be a valuable entree to the workforce. Customized workplace leaflets are one tool. An employee in contact with the single payer campaign researches the company health plan and the history of bargaining if there is a trade union there. Then she writes a leaflet with a headline like, "Prop. 186 health care without insurance companies—better than the plan at Widgets Inc." If she and a coworker can safely sign their names, they do so; if not, they identify the leaflet as coming from some employees of Widgets in favor of Proposition 186. She gets a few hundred photocopies. Workers at the company are more likely to pay attention to such a leaflet, which usually causes a stir when it appears. Because it comes from people near them and perhaps known to them, the message carries additional weight.

Customized workplace leaflets will not happen by themselves. The campaign needs to follow up with someone who volunteers to do one, just as with a house party host. Perhaps the worker wants help with editing the text. It might be necessary to recruit other people to stand utside the company entrance some morning and hand out the leaflets.

CHS filled requests from groups to send a speaker on Proposition 186, but without the priority given to fund-raising house parties. The speaker went. However, no one was responsible for investigating and following up on opportunities the group offered to reach people through its network. The campaign did not train the speaker to circulate a sign-in sheet among the audience, nor would anyone have used it afterwards. The absence of mass literature was felt at these events, too.

Building a movement through group and personal channels taps local wisdom. CHS had its natural headquarters in the San Francisco Bay Area. However, volunteers in the Los Angeles region give examples of decisions made from state headquarters, or by traveling top officials from northern California, without drawing on their knowledge and contacts. Certainly, a campaign needs central direction, but at a minimum, it would help to have local advisory committees. Unlike one person who seems like a complainer, a committee can tell headquarters and the overall steering board when it sees the job being botched. The disregard for the rich knowledge of people on the scene and the lack of well-executed decentralization testify once again to the failure to build a movement of the people.

Lesson 9: Break out of your stratum

The persons who started the initiative campaign for a single payer plan in California were mostly white, mostly men. Credit goes to them for applying their advantages of education and social position to making health care a right. Throughout the campaign its recruits were largely white people with more than average education. A large percentage of the "foot soldiers" among them were women, who remained a minority of the leading executives. Latinos and especially Black people were barely represented anywhere.

The membership of endorsing organizations was more diverse than CHS itself. But in most cases a group's endorsement consisted of the name, a donation from the treasury, and little else. However, the contrast in diversity suggests that CHS might have applied the perspective of building a movement and put resources into drawing members of trade unions and other endorsers into a mass struggle.

Obviously, the sooner that the leaders and activists of a campaign come from all strata and all parts of the working people as a whole, the sooner the campaign will have a wedge into the strata and ethnic groups themselves. However, it takes special effort to develop the wedge. Volunteers or staff must contact minority organizations with persistence to overcome their initial wariness. Somebody needs to leaflet outside unemployment offices, sifting for the person who is ready to take up the health struggle. CHS's exclusive concentration on raising money to sell a product on television prevented such efforts.

House parties, for example, mostly stayed within a narrow stratum of educated white professionals and retired people. Everyone knew this stratum combined the will and the resources to give the most money per party. By latter September the house party machine in Berkeley and Oakland overtaxed this base. Hosts found that people they invited had already attended one and even several house parties. The main direction in which CHS tried a breakout was toward the bedroom suburbs to the east.

One supporter in southern California was so upset at the lack of outreach to the Black community that she raised $3,000. With half of the money she hired a minister who appeared on radio and spoke to fellow clergymen. She spent the other half on 40,000 leaflets distributed partly by volunteers and partly by youth hired in south central Los Angeles and Pasadena. This grass roots initiative proves again how strongly people become committed to the single payer health reform, but without support from the central CHS machinery, such efforts cannot fill the void.[166]

Exit polling on election day suggested that when working people of various strata turn out, they vote in favor of Proposition 186: Latinos, 64%; uninsured people, 58%; and, confounding media talk about generation X, youth, ages 18 to 29, 62%. Campaign strategists rejected a voter registration drive because the payoff in numbers per hour of work was too low. If the campaign is not building a movement, it is true that a registration drive is uphill. The object is to start a snow-balling movement whose influx of new supporters register themselves and others. If people do not vote because they see nothing fundamental at stake, then a single payer movement has the potential of being a vital exception.

A serious campaign must solve these problems, because the stratum that initiates health reform is too small by itself to win.

Lesson 10: Realize there is no top down reform

The notion that health reform might be won from the top down is a mistaken idea held not by CHS but by national organizations. Too many trade unions, Consumers Union, and other groups put their time and energy into the Washington debate on the Clintons' plan for health alliances, Sen. Mitchell's proposal, and the trail of lesser bills that went nowhere. The problem was that there was no movement of people in the streets demanding their right. The lobbyists met with representatives in Congress armed only with brilliant policy arguments and, in some cases, simultaneous advertising on the airwaves. In an arena of money rather than masses, these groups were no match for the sections of capital that spent many tens of millions of dollars fighting to a total zero.

Consequently, when CHS out in California arrived at the headquarters of a national organization, the latter signed a paper endorsement and gave some money, at most a five-figure amount, since the six-figure allocations had already been made to national lobbying. This is one reason why trade unions, for example, did not assign significant resources in the time of paid organizers and other forms to calling out their own California members for Proposition 186, the opportunity of a lifetime to obtain health care without insurance companies and make social history.

Lesson 11: Think beyond the next milepost

The California campaign had two big mileposts: the April deadline for turning in enough signatures to qualify an initiative for the ballot, and a majority vote on Nov. 8. Either the campaign reached the goal on each of these days, or it would need to start over. Like practical people, therefore, CHS began by putting all effort into obtaining signatures, then refocused on getting votes. These were the market tests of success from the standpoint of selling a product. When building a movement, on the other hand, a campaign educates people for succeeding phases as it pursues the immediate goal.

When gathering signatures, discussion is at a minimum. The point is to maximize the count per hour of canvassing. Thinking of a movement, however, a campaign would at least supply canvassers with a half-page leaflet to be given to people who sign the petition. In California, over 600,000 signers reached by volunteers would know what they had signed, what is coming up for the election season, and whom to call to get involved.

Weren't resources a problem? CHS was $248,000 in debt on May 1, 1994. However, the leaders knew that funds would come in when the initiative qualified for the ballot, and they borrowed on that fact. The petition drive cost $830,000 including in-kind materials paid for by Neighbor to Neighbor and other coalition members. The expense of 700,000 cheap half-page leaflets is perhaps $10,000, including overhead to get them into the hands of canvassers.[167] CHS found resources to stage a pilot house party program and to take polls. In some ways, CHS did plan ahead and invest for its future, but it did not educate for the long term and build resources among the people in general.

The same thinking applied to election day. CHS dwelt on winning 50% of the votes plus one. Its strategists relied on the power of television to push the shallow waters of voting sentiment in the few days before Nov. 8. Here the failure to look beyond the next milepost is stark. If Proposition 186 loses, what has the campaign done to establish a movement that will find a way to struggle onward? Certainly, there is the core of a movement, thanks to the committed people who joined the ranks of Californians for Health Security. However, the post-election thought of CHS leaders was that the organization had a database of 25,000 names for direct mail fund raising. On the other hand, if the measure won, it would need mass support to make it a reality. The insurance corporations would have gone to court immediately, and the governor would have appointed the least vigorous person he could find to be the first health commissioner. The movement would need to stage protests in order to compel action on the people's will.

When people build a movement, they act over the long haul—which happens to be a necessity of the struggle for social justice, of which the right to health care is a part.

A Choice with a Political History

People might argue the details of these lessons, but overall the choice is between building a movement and selling a product. The CHS strategy has a political history. Saul Alinsky discovered techniques that frequently worked for small demands and short-term goals sought by community organizations, but he never came close to anything on the scope of establishing health care as a right.

Alinsky's anti-communism led him into hypocrisy that showed up his self-affixed "radical" label. In the middle of the upsurges of the late 1960s and early 1970s, he lectured, "Let us in the name of radical pragmatism not forget that in our system with all its repressions we can still speak out and denounce the administration, attack its policies, work to build an opposition political base.... That's more than I can do in Moscow, Peking, or Havana.... We have permitted a suicidal situation to unfold wherein revolution and communism have become one. These pages are committed to splitting this political atom, separating this exclusive identification of communism with revolution."[168] Since Alinsky never opposed capitalism, his talk of opening a new path to revolution was entirely phony.

Alinsky promoted a short-term outlook, a showy brand of pseudo-militancy, and fierce antagonism toward political principles. He proudly wrote, "No ideology should be more specific than that of America's founding fathers: 'For the general welfare.'"[169] Without class principles, political activity has no anchor. Inevitable drift weakens tactics, strategy, and finally the goals themselves.

Through direct personal connections, the Alinsky ideology that disclaims all ideology became one influence within the United Farm Workers Union. There is no need here to rehash the question of grape boycott and strike, or how the UFW later relied on direct mail to liberals about pesticides on food crops. Some leaders of Neighbor to Neighbor (N2N) and Californians for Health Security came out of the UFW. In the solidarity work against U.S.-supported killer regimes in Central America during the 1980s and early 1990s (the marches, the sanctuary movement, etc.), Neighbor to Neighbor's distinctive contribution was a boycott of coffee and in particular an attempt to buy television spots for it. The story of how Proctor & Gamble suppressed commercials showing Salvadoran blood dripping from a coffee cup became an issue in itself. Fascination with the modern tools of political merchandising is evident. An N2N promotional brochure tagged "Sophisticated Use of Mass Media" as one-third of its "winning combination."[170] Fortunately, nothing in the single payer plan requires this kind of politics.

More to Come

The issue of health care will not go away. Some persons in Washington know it, like Hillary Clinton. Speaking in June 1994 to the capital's Economic Club, she warned that if Congress did not enact comprehensive reform, "I can stand here and make this prediction. There will be a grassroots movement which will sweep the country that will achieve a single payer system. It will start, whether the referendum in California is successful or not. It will start there, and will build and be like nothing you have ever seen. That's what will happen."[171] Ms. Clinton is against single payer. In San Francisco on April 25, 1994, a week after backers of the California Health Security Act submitted one million signatures, she criticized a Canadian-style plan, saying, "We believe there must be a private insurance market, a mixed system between public and private financing and delivery. We like that competition."[172]

Until health care is a right, people will suffer and die. Whenever an especially tragic story hits the news, whenever Medicare is under attack, whenever new statistics show that seven or eight million Californians have no health insurance, supporters of health care without insurance companies will remind people, "With our single payer plan, this would not happen." People will fight for their right. They might win first in California, or people somewhere else might show the way. It might succeed as an issue by itself, or it might be one part of a movement now stirring below the threshold of political visibility. But it will be done. Running through the single payer movement is a struggle to decide the direction of social development as a whole. The issue of reforming health care is currently a test of our progress. Will we together watch over the health of each one of us? Will we do this as naturally as most grownups comfort a crying child? We are beginning to understand that if we as a society—not only in the family circle and in local communities—take care of each person, then we will be blessed in return with the creative and unselfish contributions of individuals to the advance of all mankind. This striving has, in the United States, come to center on the demand for health care.

Notes

1. The history of health insurance is largely taken from Lear. Survey reported on p. 209.
2. Lear, p. 214; Badger, p. 238, Rolde, p. 62.
3. Lear, p. 225.
4. Lear, p. 227.
5. Labor Research Association, 1947, p. 63.
6. Lear, p. 247.
7. Study of aged is for 1958 and reported in Gabriel Kolko, p. 118.
8. Lear, p. 229; Harmer, p. 245f.
9. Kotelchuk, p. 369f.
10. Labor Research Association, 1951, p. 54f.; National Commission to Prevent Infant Mortality, Report, 1993.
11. Nightingale quote from Rosen, p. 376; slum description from Engels, p. 66.
12. Dodd and Penrose, p. 284.
13. Nurse statistic in Buhler-Wilkerson, p. 99; *Statistical Abstract of the United States 1933*, Department of Commerce, pp. 4, 63.
14. Lear, p. 273.
15. Most of this political history comes from Badger, p. 232.
16. Frech, p. 90.
17. U.S. Dept. of Commerce, Bureau of Economic Analysis, *The National Income and Product Accounts of the United States, 1929–82: Statistical Tables*, Sept. 1986, Table 2.2. 1990 figures from *Survey of Current Business*, Aug. 1993, Table 2.6.
18. Temin, p. 76.
19. Consumers Union, p. 43.
20. 1992 statistic for private production and nonsupervisory workers, in 1982 dollars, from *Statistical Abstract 1993*, Table 667, p. 424; new job salaries from *Business Week*, July 9, 1984, p. 86; family income statistic from *Wall Street Journal*, Oct. 26, 1994, p. A2.
21. Enthoven, p. 475.
22. Census Bureau data reported in *San Francisco Chronicle*, May 26, 1994, p. A5.
23. Ginsburg, p. 188.

24. U.S. Dept. of Commerce, Bureau of Economic Analysis, *The National Income and Product Accounts of the United States, 1929–82: Statistical Tables*, Sept. 1986, Table 3.15. 1990 figures from *Survey of Current Business*, Sept. 1993, Table 3.13, p. 31.

25. Hodgson, p. 51.

26. Harmer, p. 236; Consumers Union, p. 67.

27. Temin, p. 77.

28. Reinhardt, p. 468.

29. Local 250, p. 8.

30. Starr, p. 430f, 435; *Wall Street Journal*, "Giant Hospital Chain Uses Tough Tactics To Push Fast Growth," July 12, 1994, p. A1.; *Business Week*, June 28, 1993, p. 33; Rolde, p. 33.

31. Temin, p. 78.

32. 1982 shares from Sloan, p. 103; Florida churning, Consumers Union, p. 146.

33. Local 250, p. 20ff.

34. Kotelchuk, p. 164.

35. Flexner report in Kotelchuk, p. 165, 208; 1920 meeting in Harmer, p. 18; child welfare opposition in Rosen, p. 363, 456.

36. Rosen, p. 454.

37. Rolde, p. 58.

38. Data computed from Bureau of Labor Statistics, *Handbook of Labor Statistics*, Dec. 1983, Bulletin 2175, Table 17.

39. *Statistical Abstract 1993*, Table 644, and *Monthly Labor Review*, March 1991.

40. Historical decline from Harmer, p. xiii, p. 39; current ratios from Consumers Union, p. 34.

41. Consumers Union, p. 33.

42. *Business Week*, June 8, 1992, p. 86.

43. Relman, p. 3.

44. Local 250, pp. 4, 13.

45. Local 250, pp. 6, 14.

46. Local 250, p. 4.

47. California Nurses Association, p. 7f.

48. California Nurses Association et al.

49. National Commission to Prevent Infant Mortality, Report, 1993.

50. Himmelstein, p. 76.

51. Himmelstein, p. 84.

52. Himmelstein, p. 86.

53. U.S. Dept. of Commerce, Bureau of Economic Analysis, *The National Income and Product Accounts of the United States, 1929–82: Statistical Tables*, Sept. 1986, Table 6.21B. 1990 figures from *Survey of Current Business*, Aug. 1993, Table 6.19C.

54. Relman, p. 3.

55. *San Francisco Chronicle*, April 7, 1994, p. D1.

56. *Wall Street Journal*, March 22, 1994, p. A3; *The Nation*, May 16, 1994, p. 658; Alper, p. 1523; *San Francisco Chronicle*, Dec. 8, 1994, p. A-8.

57. Harmer, p. 259; Hodgson, p. 49.

58. Kotelchuk, p. 351f.

59. Eckholm, p. 331.

60. *Business Week*, June 27, 1994, p. 32.

61. *Wall Street Journal*, April 28, 1994, p. B4.

62. *Business Week*, Sept. 19, 1994, p. 112.

63. *Business Week*, July 25, 1994, p. 88.

64. Himmelstein, p. 40.

65. Consumers Union, p. 108.

66. Kotelchuk, p. 362.

67. Woolhandler and Himmelstein, 1994, p. 265.

68. *Wall Street Journal*, May 18, 1994, p. A1.

69. Consumers Union, p. 101.

70. Oct. 10, 1993.

71. Consumers Union, p. 45.

72. HIAA, p. 23.

73. U.S. Census Bureau, *1990–1992 Survey of Income and Program Participation*, Oct. 1994.

74. Himmelstein, pp. 22, 39, 33.

75. Outcomes statistics in Consumers Union, p. 42; Harris poll in Isaacson, p. 23.

76. Consumers Union, p. 32.

77. Roemer, p. 144.

78. Most of the information on Germany is taken from Harmer and Rolde.

79. Rolde, p. 112.

80. Himmelstein, p. 114.
81. Reinhardt, p. 161.
82. Information on Sweden from Harmer and from Heclo.
83. Morton, p. 507.
84. Most of this history is from Rolde and from Harmer.
85. Himmelstein, p. 77.
86. Consumers Union, p.43.
87. *San Francisco Chronicle*, Oct. 13, 1994, p. A12.
88. Rolde, p. 129 and Himmelstein, p. 76f.
89. Harmer, p. 277.
90. Harmer, p.280.
91. Himmelstein, p. 118.
92. Consumers Union, pp. 197, 209. Most of the information about Canada is taken from Himmelstein.
93. Hospital percentages from Consumers Union, p. 47; savings calculations from Hellander, p. 4.
94. Consumers Union, p. 199.
95. *Business Week*, March 21, 1994, p. 85.
96. Himmelstein, p. 100.
97. GAO, "Canadian Health Insurance: implications for the United States," GAO/HRD–91–90, 1991.
98. Himmelstein, p. 99.
99. Himmelstein, p. 181.
100. Consumers Union, p. 201.
101. *New York Times*, Nov. 8, and Nov. 21, 1991.
102. Consumers Union, p. 220.
103. *San Francisco Chronicle*, Jan. 17, 1993.
104. Rolde, p. 206.
105. Rosko, p. 5.
106. *New York Times*, Sept. 23, 1993.
107. From a 1993 newsletter of Prudential, quoted by Himmelstein, p. 245.
108. Citizen Action research reported in *Wall Street Journal*, Feb. 4, 1994, p. A1.
109. *Wall Street Journal*, Feb. 3, 1994, p. A3.
110. Roundtable from *Wall Street Journal*, Feb. 11, 1994, p. A1; Cato Institute in *Wall Street Journal*, Feb. 14, 1994, p. A14.
111. *Wall Street Journal*, Feb. 17, 1994, p. A3.

112. *Business Week,* Nov. 28, 1994, p. 61.

113. *Wall Street Journal,* Aug. 26, 1994, p. A12.

114. *Business Week,* July 25, 1994, p. 96.

115. Newsletter to constituents. Dellums has introduced a bill for a national health service since the mid-1970s. His position for the single payer bill strengthened later in the year as the hope of reform faded.

116. Numbers refer to sections that the Act adds to the state welfare and institutions code.

117. Woolhandler and Himmelstein, 1991.

118. *New England J. of Medicine,* May 2, 1991, 234:18, p. 1254; *Health Care Financing Review,* 13:1, Fall, 1991, pp. 29–54; A. M. Best Insurance Reporting Service, 1992.

119. *San Francisco Bay Guardian,* Oct. 19, 1994, p. 27.

120. Neighbor to Neighbor, *Grounds for Action,* Summer 1993, p. 3.

121. Cohen.

122. Himmelstein, p. 198f.

123. *New York Times,* May 30, 1989, p. D1.

124. Standard & Poor's.

125. *San Francisco Bay Guardian,* Jan. 1, 1992, p. 8.

126. Company claim. Actually, with estimated 1995 California payroll figure of $1.5 billion supplied by Jean Puetz, Corporate Benefits, Hewlett-Packard, health benefits may be under 5%.

127. *New York Times,* May 30, 1989, p. D11.

128. Foner, vol. 1, p. 123.

129. Rolde, p. 7.

130. *Business Week,* Jan. 31, 1994, p. 22.

131. *Wall Street Journal,* Jan. 27, 1994, p. A2.

132. Alper, p. 1524.

133. *Wall Street Journal,* Feb. 11, 1994, p. A3.

134. *News for a People's World,* Nov. 1994, p. 3.

135. Alex Pappas.

136. Lingappa, Appendix A.

137. History of the origins of California single payer is based on interviews with Vishu Lingappa, Howard Owens and Ted Kalman.

138. Neighbor to Neighbor, *Grounds for Action,* Summer 1993, p. 1.

139. Conversation with Glen Schneider, Oct. 20, 1994.

140. *San Francisco Chronicle*, May 26, 1994, p. A5.

141. League statement of July 1994.

142. Jeanne Finberg, *California's Single Payer Initiative for Health Care: What Will it Mean for California Consumers?*, Consumers Union West Coast Regional Office, June 1994, p. 5.

143. CHS, *Yes on Prop 186: Our Winning Strategy* briefing for house party speakers, Oct. 14, 1994.

144. Pass or fail remark by Steve Schear at Vote Health meeting, July 1994; Milne quote in Butts, p. 20.

145. This writer was a speaker. The praise applies to house party speakers in general.

146. *San Francisco Examiner*, Oct. 6, 1994, and Oct. 18, 1994, p. A4; *S.F. Bay Guardian*, Oct. 19, 1994, p. 27.

147. *The Nation*, Oct. 17, 1994, p. 405.

148. *Wells Fargo Stagelines*, Oct. 1994, p. 3.

149. Dorothy P. Rice, publicly released letter to Kevin Grumbach, Aug. 25, 1994.

150. Oct. 10, 1994, p. A22.

151. *San Francisco Chronicle*, Oct. 27, 1994, p. A4.

152. *San Francisco Chronicle*, Nov. 10, 1994, p. A38.

153. *San Francisco Chronicle*, Sept. 22, 1994.

154. *San Francisco Chronicle*, Oct. 10, 1994, p. A22.

155. *New York Times*, Sept. 30, 1994, p. A9, West Coast edition.

156. Barbara Otto, SPAN, at steering committee of Californians for Health Security, Nov. 12, 1994.

157. Cloak, p. 1.

158. Speech at house party, Aug. 23, 1994.

159. Interview with Vishu Lingappa.

160. In Alameda County, immigrant defense triumphed by rejecting Proposition 187 60% to 40%. Single payer lost by 60% against to 40% in favor.

161. "Speaker's Mission & Qualifications" in the activist kit.

162. *Yes on Prop 186: Our winning strategy*, updated to Oct. 14, 1994.

163. CHS press update from Hopcraft Communications.

164. Conversation with Matthew Burry, confirmed at $2.5–2.7 million by Steve Schear.

165. Vanzetti to Judge Thayer, quoted in Read, p. 146.
166. Interview with Jo Sedita.
167. The campaign got one million signatures, but we omit leafleting by the paid canvassers who obtained 400,000 of them.
168. Alinsky, pp. xxi, 9.
169. Alinsky, p. 4.
170. *Neighbor to Neighbor: Effective Organizing* brochure. The two other tools are house meetings and helping progressive candidates get out the vote.
171. *American Health Security News*, July 1, 1994.
172. *New York Times*, April 27, 1994.

References

Alinsky, Saul D., *Rules for Radicals: A Practical Primer for Realistic Radicals*, New York, Vintage Books: Random House, 1971.

Alper, Philip R., "Primary Care in Transition," *Journal of the American Medical Association*, 272:19, Nov. 16, 1994, p. 1523.

Badger, Anthony J., *The New Deal: The Depression Years, 1933-40*, New York, Noonday Press, 1989.

Buhler-Wilkerson, Karen, "False Dawn: The Rise and Decline of Public Health Nursing in America: 1900–1930," in Ellen Condliffer Lageman, editor, *Nursing History: New Perspectives, New Possibilities*, New York, Teachers College, Columbia University, 1983, pp. 89–106.

Butts, Mickey, "California dreaming," *In These Times*, Oct. 31, 1994, p. 18.

California Nurses Association, *Big Business Means Bad Care for Bay Area Communities*, San Francisco, 1993.

California Nurses Association et al., *Alta Bates Medical Corporation: Profits Before People*, San Francisco, 1993.

Cloak, Dan, *Eight Lessons and Some Conclusions from the Single-Payer Initiative House Party Campaign*, leaflet, Nov. 11, 1994.

Cohen, Jeff, and Norman Solomon, "On the Media Beat," syndicated column, Nov. 28, 1993.

Consumers Union, *How to Resolve the Health Care Crisis: Affordable Protection for All Americans*, Yonkers, Consumer Reports Books, 1992.

Dodd, Paul A. and E. F. Penrose, *Economic Aspects of Medical Services: with special reference to California*, Washington, D.C., Graphic Arts Press, 1939.

Eckholm, Erick, ed., *Solving America's Health Care Crisis*, written by staff of *New York Times*, New York, Random House, 1993.

Engels, Frederick, *The Condition of the Working-Class in England: From Personal Observation and Authentic Sources*, Moscow, Progress Publishers, 1973.

Enthoven, Alain C., "Supply Side Economics of Health Care and Consumer Choice Health Plan," in Olson.

Finberg, Jeanne, *California's Single Payer Initiative for Health Care: What Will It Mean for California Consumers?: An Overview*, San Francisco, West Coast Regional Office of Consumers Union of U.S., Inc., June 1994.

Foner, Philip S., *History of the Labor Movement in the United States, Volume I: From Colonial Times to the Founding of the American Federation of Labor*,

New York, International Publishers, 1972.

Frech III, H. E., ed., *Health Care in America: The Political Economy of Hospitals and Health Insurance*, San Francisco, Pacific Research Institute, 1988.

Ginsburg, Paul B., "Public Insurance Programs: Medicare and Medicaid," in Frech.

Harmer, Ruth Mulvey, *American Medical Avarice*, New York, Abelard-Schuman, 1975.

Health Insurance Association of America, *Source Book of Health Insurance Data*, 1990.

Heclo, Hugh, and Henrik Madsen, *Policy and Politics in Sweden: Principled Pragmatism*, Philadelphia, Temple University Press, 1987.

Hellander, Ida et al., "Health Care Paper Chase, 1993: The Cost to the Nation, the States, and the District of Columbia," *International Journal of Health Services*, 24:1, 1994, pp. 1–9.

Himmelstein, M.D., David U., and Steffie Woolhandler, M.D., M.P.H., *The National Health Program Book: A Source Guide for Advocates*, Monroe, Maine, Common Courage Press, 1994.

Hodgson, Godfrey, "The Politics of American Health Care," *Atlantic Monthly*, Oct. 1973, p. 45.

Isaacson, Elisa, "Prescription for change," *San Francisco Bay Guardian*, April 14, 1993.

Kolko, *Gabriel, Wealth and Power in America*, New York, Praeger Publishers, 1962.

Kotelchuk, David, ed., *Prognosis Negative: Crisis in the Health Care System*, New York, Vintage, 1976.

Labor Research Association, *Labor Fact Book 8*, New York, International Publishers, 1947.

Labor Research Association, *Labor Fact Book 10*, New York, International Publishers, 1951.

Lear, M.D., Walter J., *Medical Care and Family Security*, Englewood Cliffs, N.J., Prentice-Hall, Inc., 1963.

Lingappa, Vishwanath et al, *Who do they think they are fooling? Response to the lies about Prop 186*, San Francisco, Sept. 21, 1994.

Local 250, Hospital and Health Care Works Union, SEIU, Market Share vs. Health Care: *The Hospital Council (Cartel) Helps Create A Crisis*, Oakland, 1993.

Morton, A. L., *A People's History of England*, New York, International

Publishers, 1968.

National Commission to Prevent Infant Mortality, Report, 1993.

Neighbor to Neighbor, Grounds for Action, San Francisco, Summer 1993 and Winter 1993 issues.

Olson, Mancur, ed., *A New Approach to the Economics of Health Care,* Washington, American Enterprise Institute, 1981.

Read, Herbert, *English Prose Style,* Boston, Beacon Press, 1967.

Reinhardt, Uwe, "Health Insurance and Cost Containment: The Experience Abroad," in Olson.

Relman, Arnold S., "Reforming Our Health Care System: A Physician's Perspective," *The Key Reporter,* Washington, D.C., Phi Beta Kappa, Autumn 1992.

Roemer, Milton I., *An Introduction to the U.S. Health Care System,* second edition, New York, Springer, 1986.

Rolde, Neil, *Your Money or Your Health: America's Cruel, Bureaucratic, and Horrendously Expensive Health Care System: How It Got That Way and What To Do About It,* New York, Paragon House, 1992.

Rosen, George, *A History of Public Health,* New York, MD Publications, 1958.

Rosko, Michael D. and Robert W. Broyles, *The Economics of Health Care: A Reference Handbook,* New York, Greenwood Press, 1988.

Sloan, Frank A., "Property Rights in the Hospital Industry," in Frech.

Standard & Poor's, *Register of Corporations, Directors and Executives,* New York, McGraw-Hill, 1994.

Starr, Paul, *The Social Transformation of American Medicine,* New York, Basic Books, 1982.

Temin, Peter, "An Economic History of American Hospitals," in Frech.

Woolhandler, S. and D. U. Himmelstein, "The deteriorating administrative efficiency of the U.S. health care system," *New England Journal of Medicine,* 1991, 324:1253-1258.

Woolhandler, Steffie and David U. Himmelstein, "Giant H.M.O. 'A' or Giant H.M.O. 'B'?" *The Nation,* Sept. 19, 1994, p. 265.

Index

A

AARP. *See* American Association of Retired Persons

acupuncture, 64

administrative costs, 74, 76, 92, 115

advertising. *See* marketing

Aetna Life & Casualty, 28, 29, 69, 85, 111, *113*

AFL-CIO, 92

AHA. *See* American Hospital Association

Alexander, Dan, 113

Alinsky, Saul, 104, 138

Alta Bates Corporation, 25

Alta Bates Hospital, 20-21, 97

AMA. *See* American Medical Association

American Airlines (AA), 56, 57

American Association of Retired Persons (AARP), 106, 122, 129

American College of Surgeons, 97

American Hospital Association (AHA), 12

American Medical Association (AMA), 7, 11-12, 22

Journal of, 97

American Practices Management, 24

Apple Computer, 85, 87

Association of California Life Insurance Companies, 106

B

Banks, Dwayne, 114-116

Bass family of Texas oil barons, 20

Bates, Alta Alice Miner, 21

See also Alta Bates Corporation; Alta Bates Hospital

Bauman, Robert P., 85

Baylor University, 3

Bechler, Don, 2

Bennett, William, 67

Bethlehem Steel, 56

big capital, 84-88, 103-119*passim,* 122, 123

Bismark, Otto, 38-39

Blue Cross insurance, 4, 6, 12, 17, 113

Blue Cross of California, 81

Blue Cross/Blue Shield of Massachusetts, 43

Blue Shield insurance, 5

Board of Public Health, CA, 10

Britain. *See* United Kingdom

Brown, Jerry, 25

Brown, Kathleen, 107

Budd, Edward H., 85

Business and Professions Code, 64

Business Roundtable, 55, 85-86

Business Week, 57

C

California Association of Hospitals and Health Systems, 112

California Health Security Act, 89, 91, 94, 98

See also Proposition 186